BALANCE EXERCISES FOR SENIORS

5 minutes a day to improve your balance, posture and confidence with simple home exercises to fight osteoporosis and prevent falls

ULTIMATE GUIDE

Elizabeth J. Rodgers

TABLE OF CONTENTS

CHAPTER 1: UNDERSTANDING BALANCE

Balance is a fundamental aspect of our daily lives. It allows us to walk, stand, and perform everyday activities with ease. Yet, as we age, our balance can become compromised, making us more susceptible to falls and injuries. In this chapter, we will explore the importance of balance and its impact on our overall well-being.

Balance is not just about physical stability; it is also closely linked to our posture and confidence. When we have good balance, we can maintain an upright posture, which not only improves our appearance but also supports our overall musculoskeletal health.

Good balance is the foundation for maintaining our independence and enjoying an active lifestyle. It allows us to navigate our surroundings with confidence, whether it's going for a walk in the park, climbing stairs, or engaging in our favorite hobbies.

As we age, our bodies undergo various changes that can affect our balance. Factors such as muscle weakness, joint stiffness, and changes in vision and hearing can all contribute to a decline in balance. Additionally, certain medical conditions like osteoporosis can further increase the risk of falls.

Understanding the factors that influence balance is crucial for developing effective strategies to improve it. By identifying the specific areas where we may be experiencing difficulties, we can target our efforts towards addressing those areas.

In the upcoming chapters, we will delve deeper into the various exercises and techniques that can help improve balance. We will focus on exercises that can be performed in the comfort of your own home, requiring only a few minutes of your time each day.

It's important to note that these exercises are designed to be safe and accessible for older adults. If you have any existing health conditions or concerns, it's always a good idea to consult with your healthcare provider before starting any new exercise program.

Throughout this book, we will provide detailed step-by-step instructions for each exercise, ensuring that you can perform them safely and effectively. Remember, consistency is key when it comes to improving balance. By dedicating just five minutes a day to these exercises, you can make significant progress over time.

So, let's embark on this journey together, as we explore the world of balance exercises for seniors. With each exercise, you will be one step closer to improving your balance, posture, and confidence, and ultimately, enhancing your overall quality of life.

• INTRODUCTION TO BALANCE AND STABILITY

Balance and stability are essential for maintaining independence and preventing falls as we age. In this chapter, we will explore the importance of balance and stability, and how simple exercises can help improve them. By dedicating just five minutes a day to these exercises, you can enhance your posture, boost your confidence, and reduce the risk of falls.

THE IMPORTANCE OF BALANCE AND STABILITY

Balance is the ability to maintain your body's center of gravity over its base of support. It is crucial for everyday activities such as walking, climbing stairs, and reaching for objects. As we age, our balance naturally declines due to factors like muscle weakness, joint stiffness, and changes in sensory perception.

Stability, on the other hand, refers to the ability to maintain control of your body during movement. It is closely linked to balance and plays a significant role in preventing falls. By improving your stability, you can feel more secure and confident in your movements.

The Benefits of Balance Exercises

Regular balance exercises offer numerous benefits for seniors:

- Improved Posture: Balance exercises help strengthen the muscles that support proper posture, reducing the risk of back pain and enhancing overall alignment.
- Enhanced Core Strength: Many balance exercises engage the core muscles, which are essential for stability and maintaining balance.
- Increased Flexibility: Certain balance exercises also promote flexibility, helping to maintain joint range of motion and prevent stiffness.
- Reduced Fall Risk: By improving balance and stability, you can significantly reduce the risk of falls and related injuries.
- Boosted Confidence: As you become more proficient in balance exercises, you will gain confidence in your ability to perform daily activities with ease.

Getting Started with Balance Exercises

Before starting any exercise program, it is important to consult with your healthcare provider, especially if you have any existing health conditions or concerns. Once you have the green light, you can begin incorporating balance exercises into your daily routine.

Here are a few tips to help you get started:

- Start Slow: Begin with simple exercises that you feel comfortable with, gradually increasing the difficulty as your balance improves.
- Use Support: When starting out, it can be helpful to have a sturdy chair or countertop nearby to hold onto for support.
- Focus on Form: Pay attention to your body alignment and posture during each exercise. Proper form is essential for maximizing the benefits and preventing injury.

- Be Consistent: Aim to perform balance exercises for at least five minutes a day. Consistency is key to seeing improvements in your balance and stability.

Now that you understand the importance of balance and stability and the benefits of incorporating balance exercises into your routine, it's time to dive into the specific exercises. In the next chapter, we will explore a variety of simple home exercises that target different aspects of balance and stability. Get ready to take the first step towards improving your balance, posture, and confidence!

• SYMPTOMS AND CAUSES OF BALANCE LOSS

Balance loss is a common issue among seniors and can have a significant impact on their daily lives. Understanding the symptoms and causes of balance loss is crucial in order to address the problem effectively. In this chapter, we will explore the various signs that indicate balance loss and the underlying factors that contribute to this condition.

SYMPTOMS OF BALANCE LOSS

Recognizing the symptoms of balance loss is the first step towards addressing the issue. Here are some common signs that indicate a decline in balance:

- Dizziness or lightheadedness
- Feeling unsteady or off-balance
- Difficulty walking in a straight line
- Tripping or stumbling frequently
- Having to hold onto objects or furniture for support
- Feeling like the room is spinning (vertigo)
- Experiencing frequent falls

It's important to note that experiencing one or more of these symptoms does not necessarily mean that you have a balance disorder. However, if you notice a persistent or worsening pattern, it is advisable to consult with a healthcare professional.

CAUSES OF BALANCE LOSS

Balance loss can be caused by a variety of factors, some of which are more common among seniors. Understanding the underlying causes can help in developing appropriate strategies to improve balance. Here are some of the main contributors to balance loss:

- Age-related changes: As we age, our sensory systems, such as vision, proprioception (sense of body position), and vestibular function (inner ear balance), may decline, affecting our balance.
- Muscle weakness: Weak muscles, particularly in the legs and core, can make it harder to maintain balance and stability.
- Joint stiffness: Arthritis or other joint conditions can limit range of motion and make movements more difficult, leading to balance issues.
- Medications: Certain medications can cause dizziness or affect balance, especially if they have side effects such as drowsiness or changes in blood pressure.
- Neurological conditions: Conditions like Parkinson's disease, multiple sclerosis, or stroke can impact the body's ability to maintain balance.
- Osteoporosis: Weakening of the bones due to osteoporosis can increase the risk of fractures from falls, further compromising balance.
- Other health conditions: Chronic illnesses, such as diabetes or cardiovascular disease, can affect balance indirectly by causing fatigue or affecting circulation.

It's important to note that balance loss can be influenced by a combination of these factors, and each individual may have unique circumstances contributing to their balance issues.

In the next chapter, we will delve deeper into the importance of balance exercises in addressing balance loss and preventing falls. By incorporating specific exercises into your daily routine, you can improve your balance, posture, and overall well-being.

• ASSESSING YOUR BALANCE

As we age, maintaining good balance becomes increasingly important for our overall well-being and quality of life. In this chapter, we will explore various methods to assess your balance and identify areas that may need improvement. Remember, the goal is to prevent falls and enhance your stability, which will ultimately boost your confidence and independence.

WHY ASSESS YOUR BALANCE?

Assessing your balance is the first step towards understanding your current abilities and identifying any potential areas of weakness. By evaluating your balance, you can gain insights into your posture, coordination, and stability. This assessment will help you determine the appropriate exercises and interventions needed to improve your balance and prevent falls.

SELF-ASSESSMENT

Self-assessment is a simple and effective way to gauge your balance. Here are a few exercises you can try:

1. SINGLE-LEG STANCE

Stand near a sturdy chair or countertop for support. Lift one foot off the ground and balance on the other leg. Hold this position for as long as you can, aiming for at least 30 seconds. Switch legs and repeat. Note any difficulty or wobbling during the exercise.

2. TANDEM WALK

Find a clear path in your home or outdoors. Walk heel-to-toe in a straight line, placing one foot directly in front of the other with each step. Take at least 10 steps and assess your ability to maintain balance and coordination throughout the exercise.

3. SIT-TO-STAND

Start by sitting on a sturdy chair with your feet flat on the ground. Without using your hands, stand up and then sit back down. Repeat this exercise five times and pay attention to any difficulties or instability during the transitions.

PROFESSIONAL ASSESSMENT

If you prefer a more comprehensive assessment or if you have concerns about your balance, it may be beneficial to seek a professional evaluation. A physical therapist or a healthcare provider specializing in senior fitness can conduct a thorough assessment to determine your specific needs and develop an individualized plan.

During a professional assessment, your healthcare provider may perform additional tests, such as:

1. BALANCE TESTS

These tests may involve standing on one leg, walking on different surfaces, or performing specific movements to evaluate your balance and stability. The results will help identify any areas that require improvement.

2. GAIT ANALYSIS

A gait analysis assesses your walking pattern and rhythm. By observing your gait, a healthcare professional can identify any abnormalities or issues that may contribute to balance problems.

3. STRENGTH AND FLEXIBILITY ASSESSMENT

Strength and flexibility are crucial for maintaining balance. Your healthcare provider may evaluate your muscle strength, joint mobility, and flexibility to determine how these factors impact your balance.

4. Medical History Review

During a professional assessment, your healthcare provider will review your medical history, including any previous falls or injuries, as well as any underlying conditions that may affect your balance. This information will help guide the development of your balance improvement plan.

Remember, assessing your balance is an essential first step towards improving it. By understanding your current abilities and identifying areas of weakness, you can take proactive steps to enhance your stability and prevent falls. Whether through self-assessment or a professional evaluation, the insights gained will guide your journey towards better balance and a more confident, independent lifestyle.

Chapter 2: Getting Started Safely

Welcome back! In this chapter, we will dive into the essential steps you need to take to get started safely on your balance exercise journey. It's crucial to prioritize your safety and well-being as you embark on this new chapter of your life. Let's begin!

Step 1: Consult with Your Healthcare Provider

Before starting any new exercise program, it's essential to consult with your healthcare provider, especially if you have any existing health conditions or concerns. Your doctor will provide valuable insights into any modifications or precautions you should take based on your unique circumstances. Remember, your health is our top priority!

Step 2: Create a Safe Exercise Space

Designating a safe exercise space within your home is vital for your comfort and security. Here are a few tips to help you set up your exercise area:

Clear the Clutter: Remove any obstacles or tripping hazards from the area where you plan to exercise. This includes loose rugs, cords, or any other items that may cause you to stumble.

Secure Your Space: Make sure your exercise area has stable furniture or a wall nearby that you can use for support if needed. This will provide you with an added sense of security and stability during your exercises.

Lighting Matters: Ensure that your exercise space is well-lit to minimize the risk of tripping or falling. Natural light or bright overhead lighting can make a significant difference in your safety and overall experience.

Step 3: Warm Up and Cool Down

Before and after each exercise session, it's crucial to incorporate warm-up and cool-down routines. These routines help prepare your body for exercise and prevent injury. Here's how you can do it:

Warm-Up: Begin with gentle movements such as marching in place, shoulder rolls, or ankle circles. These exercises increase blood flow to your muscles and prepare your body for the upcoming workout.

Cool-Down: After completing your exercises, take a few minutes to cool down. Perform slow, controlled movements such as stretching your arms, legs, and neck. Cooling down helps your body gradually return to its resting state and prevents dizziness or lightheadedness.

Step 4: Start Slow and Progress Gradually

Remember, Rome wasn't built in a day, and neither will your balance and stability. It's essential to start slow and gradually increase the difficulty of your exercises over time. Here's how you can do it:

Set Realistic Goals: Begin with achievable goals that align with your current fitness level. For example, aim to perform each exercise for a specific duration or complete a certain number of repetitions. As you build strength and confidence, you can gradually increase these goals.

Listen to Your Body: Pay close attention to how your body feels during and after each exercise. If you experience pain or discomfort, it's essential to modify the exercise or seek guidance from your healthcare provider. Your body knows best!

Step 5: Stay Consistent and Motivated

Consistency is key when it comes to reaping the benefits of balance exercises. Here are a few tips to help you stay motivated and committed to your exercise routine:

Find an Accountability Partner: Partner up with a friend or family member who can join you in your exercise journey. Having someone to share your progress and challenges with can provide the motivation and support you need.

Track Your Progress: Keep a journal or use a fitness app to track your progress. Celebrate each milestone, no matter how small, and use these achievements as fuel to keep going.

Make It Enjoyable: Find ways to make your exercise routine enjoyable. Listen to your favorite music, watch a TV show, or even dance while you exercise. Making it fun will help you look forward to your daily balance exercises.

That's it for Chapter 2! By following these steps, you are setting yourself up for success in your balance exercise journey. Remember, safety and consistency are the pillars of your progress. In the next chapter, we will explore specific balance exercises that will help improve your posture and stability. Get ready to take the next step towards a healthier, more confident you!

• PREPARING YOURSELF FOR EXERCISE

As we embark on this journey of improving your balance, posture, and confidence, it is crucial to prepare yourself for exercise. This chapter will guide you through the necessary steps to ensure you are physically and mentally ready to begin your balance exercises.

1. CONSULT YOUR HEALTHCARE PROVIDER

Before starting any exercise program, it is essential to consult with your healthcare provider, especially if you have any pre-existing health conditions or concerns. Your healthcare provider will be able to assess your current health status and provide personalized recommendations.

2. CREATE A SAFE EXERCISE SPACE

Designating a safe and comfortable area in your home for your balance exercises is crucial. Clear any obstacles or clutter that may pose a tripping hazard, and ensure there is enough space to move freely. Consider using a non-slip mat or rug to provide stability during your exercises.

3. GATHER NECESSARY EQUIPMENT

Most of the balance exercises in this book require little to no equipment. However, having a sturdy chair or countertop nearby for support can be helpful, especially if you are just starting or have concerns about your balance. Additionally, keep a water bottle nearby to stay hydrated throughout your exercise routine.

4. DRESS COMFORTABLY

Wearing comfortable, non-restrictive clothing and supportive footwear is essential for optimal performance and safety during your balance exercises. Choose clothing that allows you to move freely and shoes that provide stability and traction.

5. WARM-UP AND COOL DOWN

Before and after each exercise session, it is important to warm up and cool down your muscles. This helps prevent injury and prepares your body for the upcoming exercises. A simple warm-up can include gentle movements such as marching in place or shoulder rolls. Cooling down can be as simple as taking a few deep breaths and stretching your muscles.

6. LISTEN TO YOUR BODY

Pay attention to your body's signals during your balance exercises. If you experience pain, dizziness, or shortness of breath, stop the exercise and rest. It is normal to feel some muscle fatigue, but pushing through sharp or intense pain is not recommended. Take breaks as needed and gradually increase the intensity and duration of your exercises over time.

7. STAY CONSISTENT

Consistency is key when it comes to reaping the benefits of balance exercises. Aim to incorporate these exercises into your daily routine, even if it's just for a few minutes.

Remember, it's better to do a little bit every day than to do a lot once in a while. Set realistic goals and track your progress to stay motivated and accountable.

By following these steps and preparing yourself for exercise, you are setting yourself up for success on your journey to improved balance, posture, and confidence. Now, let's dive into the first set of balance exercises in the next chapter!

• SAFETY CONSIDERATIONS AND PRECAUTIONS

When engaging in any exercise routine, it is essential to prioritize safety to prevent injuries. This chapter will outline some important safety considerations and precautions that you should keep in mind while performing the balance exercises in this book. By following these guidelines, you can ensure a safe and effective workout that promotes your overall well-being.

CONSULT YOUR HEALTHCARE PROVIDER

Before starting any new exercise program, it is crucial to consult with your healthcare provider, especially if you have any pre-existing health conditions or concerns. They can provide personalized advice and guidance based on your unique circumstances.

It is particularly important to seek medical advice if you have a history of falls, osteoporosis, or any other musculoskeletal issues. Your healthcare provider will be able to assess your current physical condition and determine if there are any specific exercises or modifications that you should consider.

START SLOW AND PROGRESS GRADUALLY

When beginning a new exercise routine, it is important to start slow and progress gradually. This approach allows your body to adapt to the exercises and reduces the risk of overexertion or injury.

Begin with the introductory exercises provided in this book, focusing on proper form and technique. As you become more comfortable and confident, you can gradually increase the intensity or duration of the exercises. Listen to your body and avoid pushing yourself too hard too soon.

USE PROPER EQUIPMENT

Using the right equipment is essential for maintaining safety during your balance exercises.

Wear comfortable, supportive shoes that provide stability and grip. Avoid exercising in socks or barefoot, as this can increase the risk of slipping or falling. Additionally, consider using a sturdy chair or wall for support during certain exercises, especially if you have concerns about balance.

MODIFY EXERCISES AS NEEDED

It is important to remember that everyone's fitness level and physical capabilities are different.

If you find that certain exercises are too challenging or cause discomfort, don't hesitate to modify them to suit your needs. For example, you can reduce the range of motion, decrease the number of repetitions, or use additional support if necessary. The key is to listen to your body and make adjustments that allow you to perform the exercises safely and comfortably.

PAY ATTENTION TO WARNING SIGNS

During your balance exercises, it is crucial to pay attention to any warning signs that indicate potential issues.

If you experience dizziness, shortness of breath, chest pain, or any other concerning symptoms, stop exercising immediately and seek medical attention. These symptoms may be indicative of an underlying health condition or overexertion.

Additionally, if you feel any sharp or intense pain during an exercise, stop and assess the situation. It is normal to feel some muscle soreness or fatigue, but sharp or intense pain should not be ignored.

STAY HYDRATED

Proper hydration is essential for optimal exercise performance and overall health. Make sure to drink water before, during, and after your balance exercises to stay hydrated. Dehydration can lead to fatigue, dizziness, and other complications, so it is important to prioritize hydration throughout your workout.

Remember, these safety considerations and precautions are meant to ensure your well-being while performing the balance exercises in this book. By following these guidelines, you can minimize the risk of injuries and maximize the benefits of your exercise routine. Always prioritize your safety and listen to your body throughout the process.

• IMPORTANCE OF PROPER BREATHING TECHNIQUES

Proper breathing techniques are essential for overall health and well-being, especially for seniors. In this chapter, we will explore the importance of breathing correctly and how it can positively impact balance, posture, and confidence.

THE CONNECTION BETWEEN BREATHING AND BALANCE

Did you know that your breath can affect your balance? It may seem surprising, but the way you breathe can influence your body's stability. When you take shallow breaths or hold your breath, it can create tension and stiffness in your muscles, making it harder to maintain your balance. On the other hand, deep and controlled breathing can help relax your body and improve your ability to stay steady on your feet.

One of the main reasons proper breathing is crucial for balance is its impact on the core muscles. Your core muscles, including the abdominal and back muscles, play a significant role in maintaining stability and good posture. When you breathe deeply and engage your diaphragm, these muscles are activated, providing support and stability to your spine and pelvis. This, in turn, enhances your overall balance and reduces the risk of falls.

THE BENEFITS OF DEEP BREATHING

Deep breathing, also known as diaphragmatic breathing or belly breathing, offers numerous benefits for seniors. Let's explore some of the advantages:

- Improved Oxygenation: Deep breathing increases the amount of oxygen in your bloodstream, promoting better overall health and vitality.
- Reduced Stress and Anxiety: Deep breathing triggers the relaxation response in your body, helping to calm your mind and reduce stress and anxiety.
- Enhanced Posture: Deep breathing encourages proper alignment of the spine, which can improve your posture and prevent slouching.
- Increased Focus and Concentration: By bringing your attention to your breath, deep breathing can help improve your concentration and mental clarity.
- Improved Digestion: Deep breathing stimulates the parasympathetic nervous system, which promotes optimal digestion and absorption of nutrients.

SIMPLE BREATHING EXERCISES FOR SENIORS

Now that you understand the importance of proper breathing, let's explore some simple breathing exercises that can help improve your balance, posture, and overall well-being.

DEEP BELLY BREATHING:

Find a comfortable seated position with your feet flat on the floor. Place one hand on your belly and the other on your chest. Take a slow, deep breath in through your nose, allowing your belly to rise as you fill your lungs with air. Exhale slowly through your mouth, feeling your belly fall. Repeat this deep belly breathing for several minutes, focusing on the sensation of your breath moving in and out of your body.

4-4-6 BREATHING:

This breathing technique can help you relax and reduce stress. Sit or lie down in a comfortable position. Close your eyes and take a deep breath in through your nose for a count of 4. Hold your breath for a count of 4. Exhale slowly through your mouth for a count of 6. Repeat this cycle for several rounds, gradually increasing the duration of each count as you become more comfortable.

HUMMING BREATH:

This exercise can help improve lung capacity and promote relaxation. Sit comfortably and take a deep breath in through your nose. As you exhale, make a humming sound, feeling the vibrations in your throat. Continue to inhale deeply and exhale with a humming sound for several breaths.

TRIANGLE BREATHING:

This technique can help improve focus and concentration. Imagine a triangle in your mind. Inhale slowly as you trace one side of the triangle in your mind. Hold your breath as you trace the second side. Exhale slowly as you trace the third side. Repeat this triangle breathing pattern for several rounds, focusing on the visualization of the triangle as you breathe.

Remember, consistency is key when it comes to reaping the benefits of these breathing exercises. Aim to incorporate them into your daily routine, even if it's just for a few minutes a day. As you practice these techniques regularly, you'll notice improvements in your balance, posture, and overall confidence.

Take a moment now to try one of the breathing exercises mentioned above. Close your eyes, take a deep breath, and let the rhythm of your breath guide you towards a greater sense of balance and well-being.

CHAPTER 3: SEATED EXERCISES

Welcome to Chapter 3, a pivotal section of our journey toward improved balance, stability, and overall well-being. As we age, maintaining balance becomes increasingly important in our daily lives. It's not just about avoiding falls—although that's certainly a critical aspect—but also about enhancing our confidence, posture, and the ability to move through the world with ease. This chapter focuses on **seated exercises**, which are designed to help you strengthen your body and improve your balance without the need to stand or put weight on your legs.

These exercises are gentle, accessible, and specifically tailored to seniors who may have limited mobility or are at a higher risk of falls. By incorporating these exercises into your daily routine, you'll be taking proactive steps to enhance your stability, boost your confidence, and support your overall health.

THE IMPORTANCE OF SEATED EXERCISES

For many seniors, traditional standing exercises may feel daunting or unsafe, particularly if balance has already become a concern. **Seated exercises** offer a safe and effective alternative. By performing these exercises while seated, you can focus on building strength, improving coordination, and enhancing flexibility without the risk of falling. Additionally, seated exercises are an excellent way to engage muscles that are essential for balance and stability, such as your core, legs, and lower back, all while minimizing strain on your joints.

Seated exercises are also highly adaptable. Whether you're dealing with arthritis, recovering from an injury, or simply prefer a lower-impact workout, these exercises can be easily modified to meet your individual needs. The key is consistency—regular practice will help you build strength and stability over time, leading to better balance and a reduced risk of falls.

WHAT YOU'LL LEARN IN THIS CHAPTER

This chapter introduces a variety of exercises that you can perform from the comfort of a sturdy chair. Each exercise is designed to target specific muscle groups that contribute to overall balance and stability. Let's take a closer look at what you'll be doing:

1. **Seated Marching:** This exercise is a great way to start your routine. It involves lifting your feet off the ground in a marching motion, which helps to activate the muscles in your legs and improve coordination. It's a simple yet effective way to warm up and get your blood flowing.

2. **Seated Leg Extensions:** By extending your legs out in front of you, you'll engage your quadriceps—the large muscles on the front of your thighs. Strengthening these muscles is essential for maintaining stability, especially when walking or standing up from a seated position.

3. **Seated Heel and Toe Raises:** This exercise focuses on your calf muscles and ankles, both of which play a crucial role in balance. By lifting your heels and toes alternately, you'll improve the strength and stability of your lower legs, helping to prevent falls.

4. **Seated Upper Body Twist:** Twisting your upper body while keeping your hips stable is a fantastic way to enhance your core stability and improve the mobility of your spine. A strong core is vital for maintaining balance and posture, making this exercise particularly beneficial.

5. **Seated Shoulder Rolls:** This exercise is designed to relieve tension in your shoulders and upper back, areas that often become tight due to poor posture or stress. By rolling your shoulders in a circular motion, you'll improve flexibility and promote better posture.

6. **Seated Abdominal Contractions:** Engaging your abdominal muscles is key to building a strong core. This exercise involves contracting your abs, which helps to strengthen the muscles that support your spine and contribute to overall balance.

7. **Seated Neck Stretches:** Often overlooked, the muscles in your neck play a significant role in your overall well-being. Stretching these muscles can help to alleviate tension, improve flexibility, and support better posture.

THE BENEFITS OF SEATED EXERCISES

The benefits of incorporating seated exercises into your routine are numerous and far-reaching. Here are some of the key advantages:

1. **Improved Balance and Stability:** By regularly engaging in these exercises, you'll strengthen the muscles that are critical for maintaining balance, both when you're seated and when you're moving about.

2. **Enhanced Posture:** Poor posture can lead to a host of issues, including back pain and reduced mobility. The exercises in this chapter will help you develop a stronger core, which in turn will support better posture.

3. **Reduced Risk of Falls:** Falls are a major concern for seniors, often leading to serious injuries. By improving your balance and strengthening your muscles, you'll significantly reduce your risk of falling.

4. **Increased Confidence:** As you build strength and stability, you'll likely notice a boost in your confidence. Moving through your day with greater ease and assurance can have a positive impact on your overall quality of life.

5. **Flexibility and Range of Motion:** Many of the exercises in this chapter focus on stretching and improving the flexibility of key muscle groups. This can lead to a greater range of motion, making everyday tasks easier and more comfortable.

6. **Stress Relief and Relaxation:** Seated exercises are not just about physical strength—they also offer an opportunity to relax and relieve stress. Many of the

exercises include elements of deep breathing and mindfulness, which can help to calm your mind and reduce tension.

REASSURANCE AND ENCOURAGEMENT

As you embark on this chapter, it's important to remember that progress takes time. The exercises outlined here are designed to be simple and easy to follow, even for those who are new to exercise or who may be dealing with physical limitations. The key to success is consistency—by practicing these exercises regularly, you'll gradually build strength and stability.

Don't be discouraged if you find some exercises challenging at first. It's perfectly normal to start slowly and gradually increase the intensity as you become more comfortable. The most important thing is to listen to your body and proceed at a pace that feels right for you. If you experience any discomfort or pain, stop the exercise and consult with a healthcare professional.

Remember, these exercises are designed to be gentle and accessible. There's no need to rush or push yourself too hard. The goal is to improve your balance and stability over time, so be patient and give yourself the space to progress at your own pace.

COMMITMENT AND CONSISTENCY

To reap the full benefits of these seated exercises, it's essential to make them a regular part of your routine. Aim to incorporate these exercises into your daily life, whether it's first thing in the morning, during a break in the afternoon, or as part of your evening wind-down. The more consistently you practice, the more you'll notice improvements in your balance, posture, and overall well-being.

By committing to these exercises, you're taking an important step towards maintaining your independence, reducing your risk of falls, and improving your quality of life. Each time you complete a session, you're investing in your health and your future.

In conclusion, this chapter is your guide to improving balance and stability from the comfort of your chair. With simple, effective exercises that are easy to follow, you have the tools you need to enhance your well-being and enjoy greater confidence in your daily life. So, take a deep breath, find a comfortable seat, and let's get started on the path to better balance and a healthier you!

• GENTLE EXERCISES TO IMPROVE STABILITY FROM A SEATED POSITION

Welcome to the chapter on gentle exercises to improve stability from a seated position. These exercises are specifically designed to help seniors enhance their balance and stability while sitting, making them accessible to individuals with limited mobility. By incorporating these exercises into your daily routine, you can strengthen your core muscles, improve posture, and reduce the risk of falls.

EXERCISE 1: SEATED MARCHING

Start by sitting upright in a sturdy chair with your feet flat on the floor. Place your hands on your thighs for support. Lift one foot off the ground and march in place, bringing your knee up towards your chest. Lower your foot back down and repeat with the other leg. Aim for 10 to 15 repetitions on each side. This exercise helps to activate the muscles in your legs and improve coordination.

EXERCISE 6: SITTING SIDE TILT

This is a great exercise to begin with because it warms up the body while improving core strength. Sit up straight in your chair and tilt your upper body as far as you can to the lef to center, then repeat the exercise on your right.

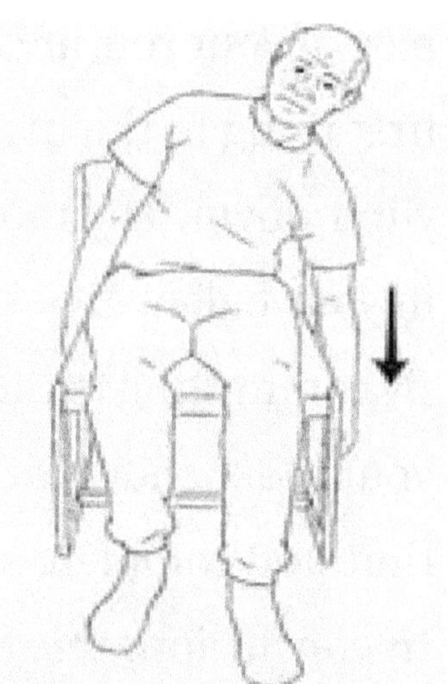

EXERCISE 2: SEATED HEEL AND TOE RAISES

Sit with your feet flat on the floor, hip-width apart. Lift your heels off the ground, keeping your toes on the floor. Hold for a few seconds and then lower your heels back down. Next, lift your toes off the ground while keeping your heels down. Hold for a few seconds and then lower your toes back down. Repeat this sequence 10 to 15 times. These exercises help strengthen your calf muscles and improve ankle stability.

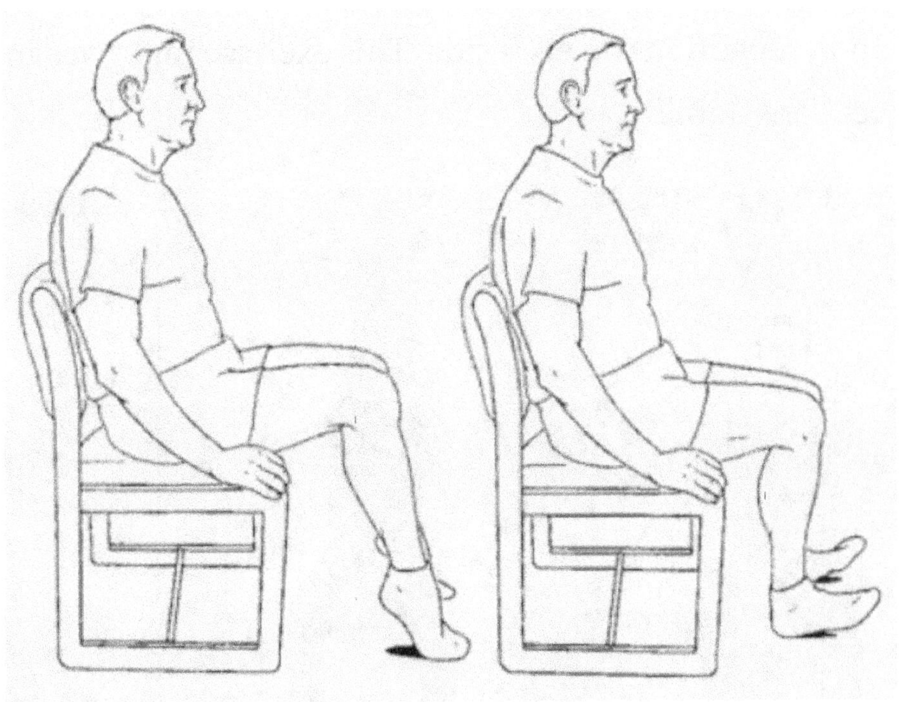

EXERCISE 3: SEATED SHOULDER ROLLS

Sit upright with your feet flat on the floor and relax your arms by your sides. Roll your shoulders forward in a circular motion, starting with small circles and gradually increasing the size. After a few rotations, reverse the direction and roll your shoulders backward. Perform 10 to 15 repetitions in each direction. This exercise helps to relieve tension in your shoulders and upper back, promoting better posture.

EXERCISE 5: SEATED NECK STRETCHES

Sit with your back straight and feet flat on the floor. Gently tilt your head to the right, bringing your right ear towards your right shoulder. Hold for a few seconds and then return to the center. Repeat the stretch to the left side. Perform 5 to 10 repetitions on each side. This exercise helps to alleviate tension in your neck and improve flexibility.

EXERCISE 4: SEATED UPPER BODY TWIST

Sit tall with your feet flat on the floor and place your hands on your shoulders. Slowly twist your upper body to the right, keeping your hips and lower body stable. Hold for a few seconds and then return to the starting position. Repeat the twist to the left side. Aim for 10 to 15 repetitions on each side. This exercise improves mobility in your spine and enhances core stability.

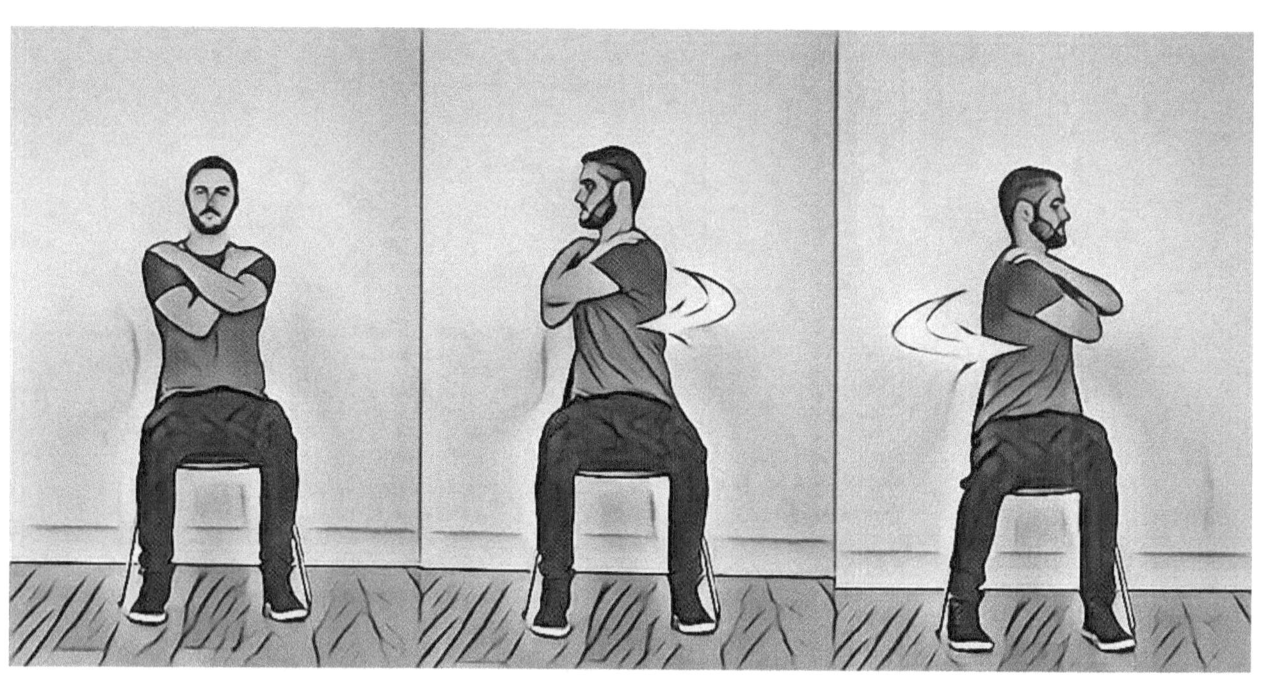

EXERCISE7: SEATED ABDOMINAL CONTRACTIONS

Sit tall with your feet flat on the floor and place your hands on your thighs. Take a deep breath in and as you exhale, gently draw your belly button towards your spine, engaging your abdominal muscles. Hold for a few seconds and then release. Repeat this contraction 10 to 15 times. This exercise strengthens your core muscles, which are essential for maintaining stability and balance.

Remember to perform these exercises in a slow and controlled manner, focusing on proper form and breathing throughout. If you experience any pain or discomfort during the exercises, stop immediately and consult with a healthcare professional.

By incorporating these gentle exercises into your daily routine, you can improve your stability, posture, and overall well-being. Stay committed and consistent, and you will gradually notice the benefits of these simple yet effective exercises. Take charge of your health and enjoy the freedom and confidence that comes with improved balance!

• CHAIR EXERCISES AND STRETCHING ROUTINES

As we continue reading this chapter, in addition to exploring the series of chair exercises we have seen before and will repeat again now, we also add those stretching routines designed specifically to improve balance and flexibility. These exercises can be easily performed at home, using a sturdy chair for support.

CHAIR EXERCISES & STRETCHING ROUTINES

1. Shoulder Stretch: Sit upright in a chair with your feet flat on the floor. Reach your right arm across your chest, placing your left hand on your right elbow. Gently pull your right arm towards your chest, feeling a stretch in your shoulder. Hold this stretch for 15-30 seconds, then switch sides. This stretch helps to release tension in the shoulders and improve range of motion.

2. Hamstring Stretch: Sit upright in a chair with your feet flat on the floor. Extend one leg straight out in front of you, keeping your heel on the ground. Lean forward from your hips, reaching towards your toes. Hold this stretch for 15-30 seconds, then switch legs. This stretch targets the muscles in the back of your thighs and helps to improve flexibility.

3. Seated Leg Extensions: Seated leg extensions are a seated exercise that helps to strengthen the quadriceps muscles in the front of the thighs.

- Sit on a chair with your feet flat on the floor and your back straight.

- Extend one leg out in front of you, straightening your knee as much as you can.

- Hold for a few seconds, then lower your leg back down.

- Repeat the exercise with the other leg, alternating legs for 10 repetitions.

- Rest for 15 seconds, then complete 2 more sets of 10 repetitions, resting for 15 seconds between each set.

Important: Keep your core engaged and maintain good posture throughout the exercise. If you have difficulty balancing, you can hold onto the sides of the chair for support.

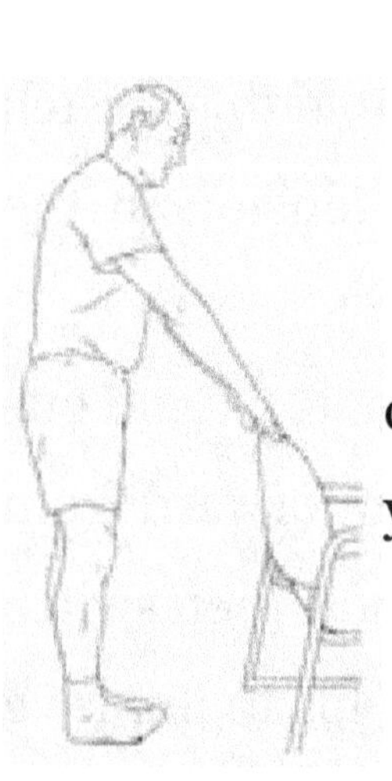

9. ANKLE BEND

This exercise primarily works to improve your balance. Holding your chair for support, press your left heel into the floor and gently bend your ankle and raise your toes, keeping your body straight throughout the exercise. Lower your toes and repeat with right leg.

Remember: Before starting any exercise program, it's important to consult with your healthcare provider, especially if you have any pre-existing health conditions or concerns. Listen to your body and only perform exercises that feel comfortable and safe for you. If you experience any pain or discomfort during an exercise, stop immediately and seek medical advice.

That concludes Chapter 3 of "Balance Exercises for Seniors: 5 minutes a day to improve your balance, posture, and confidence with simple home exercises to fight osteoporosis and prevent falls." These chair exercises and stretching routines are a great way to improve your balance and flexibility from the comfort of your own home. Stay tuned for the next chapter, where we will explore additional exercises to further enhance your stability and overall well-being.

• BREATHING AND RELAXATION TECHNIQUES

As we continue our journey towards better balance and posture, it's important to remember that our breath plays a crucial role in maintaining our overall well-being. In this chapter, we will explore breathing and relaxation techniques that can help you improve your balance and enhance your sense of calm and focus.

THE POWER OF BREATH

Take a moment to notice your breath. Is it shallow or deep? Fast or slow? Our breath is not only essential for our survival but also has a profound impact on our physical and mental state. By practicing deep, mindful breathing, we can activate the relaxation response in our body, reducing stress and promoting a sense of calm.

DIAPHRAGMATIC BREATHING

One effective breathing technique for relaxation and balance is diaphragmatic breathing, also known as belly breathing. This technique involves breathing deeply into your diaphragm, allowing your belly to rise and fall with each breath.

To practice diaphragmatic breathing:

- Find a comfortable seated position, with your feet flat on the floor and your spine straight.
- Place one hand on your chest and the other on your belly.

- Inhale slowly through your nose, allowing your belly to rise as you fill your lungs with air.

- Exhale slowly through your mouth, feeling your belly gently contract as you release the breath.

- Repeat this deep, slow breathing pattern for several minutes, focusing on the sensation of your breath moving in and out of your body.

Diaphragmatic breathing can help you relax your muscles, reduce tension, and improve your overall sense of balance and well-being.

MINDFUL BREATHING

In addition to diaphragmatic breathing, practicing mindfulness can further enhance your balance and relaxation. Mindful breathing involves bringing your full attention to the present moment and observing your breath without judgment.

To practice mindful breathing:

- Find a quiet, comfortable space where you can sit or lie down.

- Close your eyes and take a few deep breaths, allowing your body to relax.

- Shift your focus to your breath, noticing the sensation of the air entering and leaving your body.

- As thoughts or distractions arise, gently acknowledge them without judgment and bring your attention back to your breath.

- Continue this practice for several minutes, allowing yourself to fully immerse in the present moment.

Mindful breathing can help improve your concentration, reduce stress, and enhance your overall sense of balance and well-being.

PROGRESSIVE MUSCLE RELAXATION

Another technique to promote relaxation and improve balance is progressive muscle relaxation. This technique involves systematically tensing and releasing different muscle groups to release tension and promote a sense of calm.

To practice progressive muscle relaxation:

- Find a comfortable position, either sitting or lying down.
- Starting with your toes, tense the muscles in that area for a few seconds, then release and let them relax completely.
- Move up to your feet, calves, thighs, and continue tensing and releasing each muscle group.
- Work your way up your body, including your abdomen, chest, arms, shoulders, neck, and face.
- Take your time with each muscle group, focusing on the sensation of tension and relaxation.

Progressive muscle relaxation can help release physical tension, improve body awareness, and enhance your overall sense of balance and well-being.

THE BENEFITS OF RELAXATION TECHNIQUES

By incorporating breathing and relaxation techniques into your daily routine, you can experience a wide range of benefits:

- Reduced stress and anxiety
- Improved sleep quality
- Enhanced focus and concentration
- Increased self-awareness
- Improved emotional well-being
- Enhanced balance and posture
- Reduced muscle tension and pain

Remember, these techniques are not just limited to your exercise routine. You can practice them anytime, anywhere, to bring a sense of calm and balance to your daily life.

Take a moment now to try one of the techniques mentioned above. Close your eyes, take a deep breath, and allow yourself to fully immerse in the experience. Notice how your body and mind respond to the practice. With regular practice, you can harness the power of your breath to improve your balance, posture, and overall well-being.

Chapter 4: Standing Strong

In this chapter, we will focus on exercises that will help you stand strong and improve your balance. By incorporating these exercises into your daily routine, you will build strength in your legs and core, which are essential for maintaining stability and preventing falls.

Before we dive into the exercises, let's take a moment to understand why standing strong is so important. As we age, our muscles naturally weaken, and our sense of balance may decline. This combination puts us at a higher risk of falling, which can lead to serious injuries. By practicing these exercises regularly, you can strengthen your muscles, improve your balance, and reduce the risk of falls.

- **Techniques to Enhance Posture and Stability**

The Tree Pose

This exercise is inspired by the graceful stance of a tree, and it helps improve your balance and stability. Find a quiet space in your home where you can stand comfortably. Begin by standing tall with your feet together and your arms relaxed by your sides. Take a deep breath in, and as you exhale, shift your weight onto your left foot. Slowly lift your right foot off the ground, bending your knee and placing the sole of your right foot against your left leg, either below or above the knee. Find a spot in front of you to focus on, which will help with your balance. Once you feel stable, bring your hands together in front of your chest, like you're holding a prayer. Hold this pose for 30 seconds to 1 minute, focusing on your breath and maintaining your balance. Slowly release the pose and repeat on the other side.

Important: If you find it challenging to maintain your balance in this pose, you can use a wall or a chair for support. Place your fingertips lightly on the wall or hold onto the back of the chair to help you stay steady. As you practice, you'll gradually build strength and stability, allowing you to perform the pose without support.

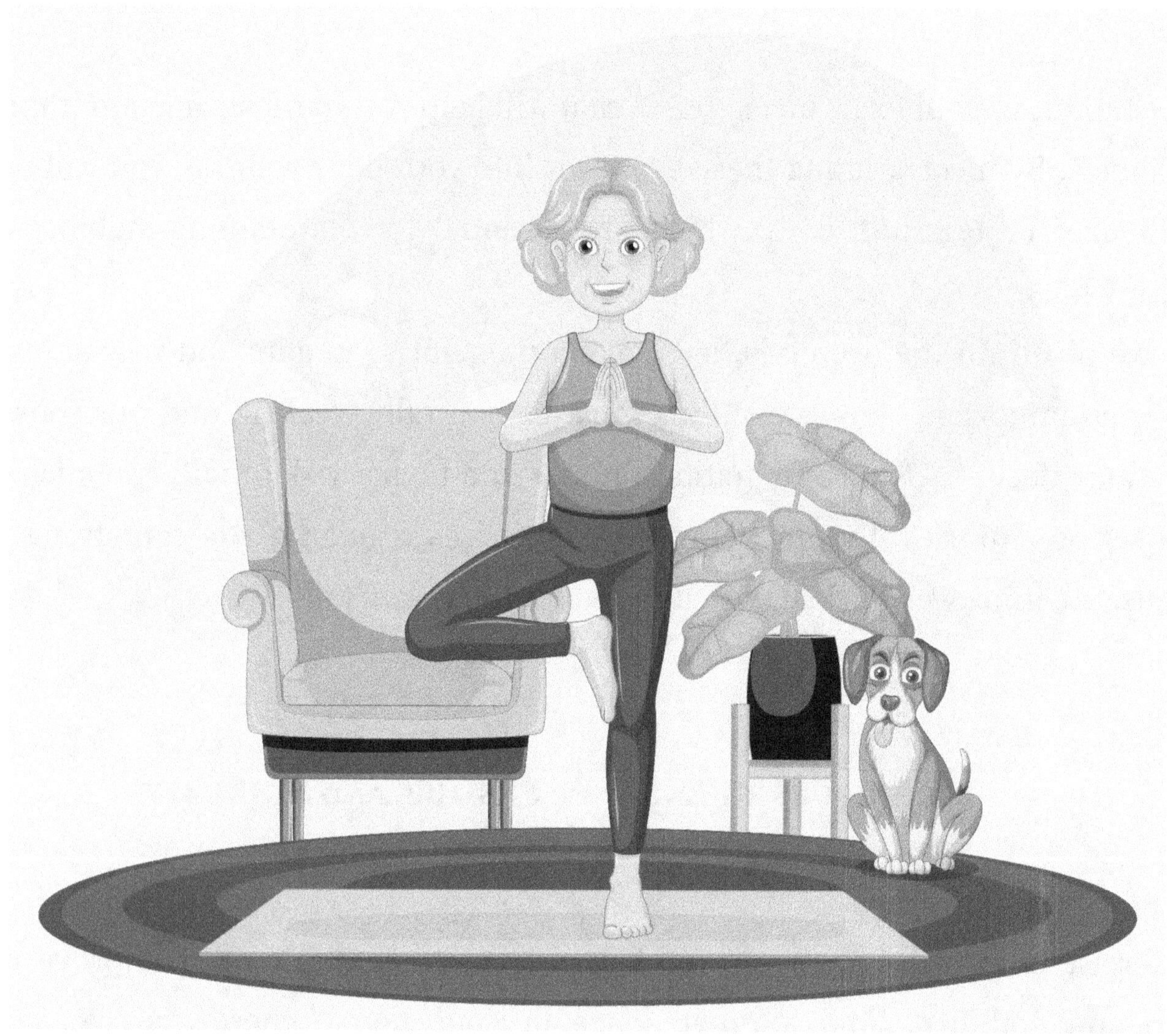

THE HEEL-TO-TOE WALK

This exercise is a simple yet effective way to improve your balance and coordination. Find a clear path in your home where you can walk in a straight line. Stand tall with your feet together, and take a deep breath in. As you exhale, take a step forward by placing your right heel directly in front of your left toe. Your right foot should be touching the heel of your left foot. Take another step forward, this time bringing your left heel to touch the toe of your right foot. Continue walking in this heel-to-toe pattern for 10 to 15 steps. As you walk, focus on keeping your gaze forward and your posture upright. This exercise challenges your balance and works your leg muscles, helping you build strength and stability.

Important: If you feel unsteady while performing this exercise, you can place your hand on a wall or a piece of furniture for support. As you gain confidence and improve your balance, try to wean off the support and perform the exercise without assistance.

THE SINGLE LEG STAND

This exercise is a great way to strengthen your leg muscles and improve your balance. Find a clear space in your home where you can stand comfortably. Begin by standing tall with your feet hip-width apart and your arms relaxed by your sides. Take a deep breath in, and as you exhale, shift your weight onto your left foot. Slowly lift your right foot off the ground, bending your knee and bringing it up towards your chest. Find a spot in front of you to focus on, which will help with your balance. Hold this position for 10 to 30 seconds, depending on your comfort level. Slowly lower your right foot back down to the ground and repeat on the other side.

Important: If you find it challenging to maintain your balance in this exercise, you can use a wall or a chair for support. Place your fingertips lightly on the wall or hold onto the back of the chair to help you stay steady. As you practice, you'll gradually build strength and stability, allowing you to perform the exercise without support.

Remember, consistency is key when it comes to improving your balance and strength. Aim to incorporate these exercises into your daily routine, starting with just a few minutes a day and gradually increasing the duration as you feel more comfortable. By dedicating a few minutes each day to these exercises, you'll be taking a proactive step towards maintaining your independence, preventing falls, and enhancing your overall well-being.

To continue our journey toward better balance and stability, it is time to explore strengthening exercises that can be performed while standing. These exercises target the leg, core and upper body muscles and help improve overall balance and prevent falls. Remember that consistency is key, so try to perform these exercises for just five minutes a day to see significant improvements in balance, posture and confidence. Some you already know but it is good to perform them again, others will be new exercises to do to feel better

1. SIDE LEG LIFT

The side leg lift exercise targets the muscles in your hips and outer thighs, which play a crucial role in maintaining balance. To perform this exercise:

- Stand up straight with your feet hip-width apart and your hands resting on a sturdy surface for support.
- Shift your weight onto your left leg.
- Lift your right leg out to the side, keeping it straight and your toes pointing forward.
- Lower your right leg back down to the starting position.
- Repeat this exercise for 10-15 repetitions on each leg.

Important: Focus on maintaining proper form and avoid leaning or tilting your upper body while performing this exercise.

2. STANDING CALF RAISES

The standing calf raises exercise targets the muscles in your calves, which are essential for maintaining balance and stability. To perform this exercise:

- Stand up straight with your feet hip-width apart and your hands resting on a sturdy surface for support.

- Raise your heels off the ground, lifting your body up onto the balls of your feet.

- Hold this position for a few seconds, then lower your heels back down to the starting position.

- Repeat this exercise for 10-15 repetitions.

Important: If you need additional support, you can perform this exercise while standing near a wall or holding onto a chair.

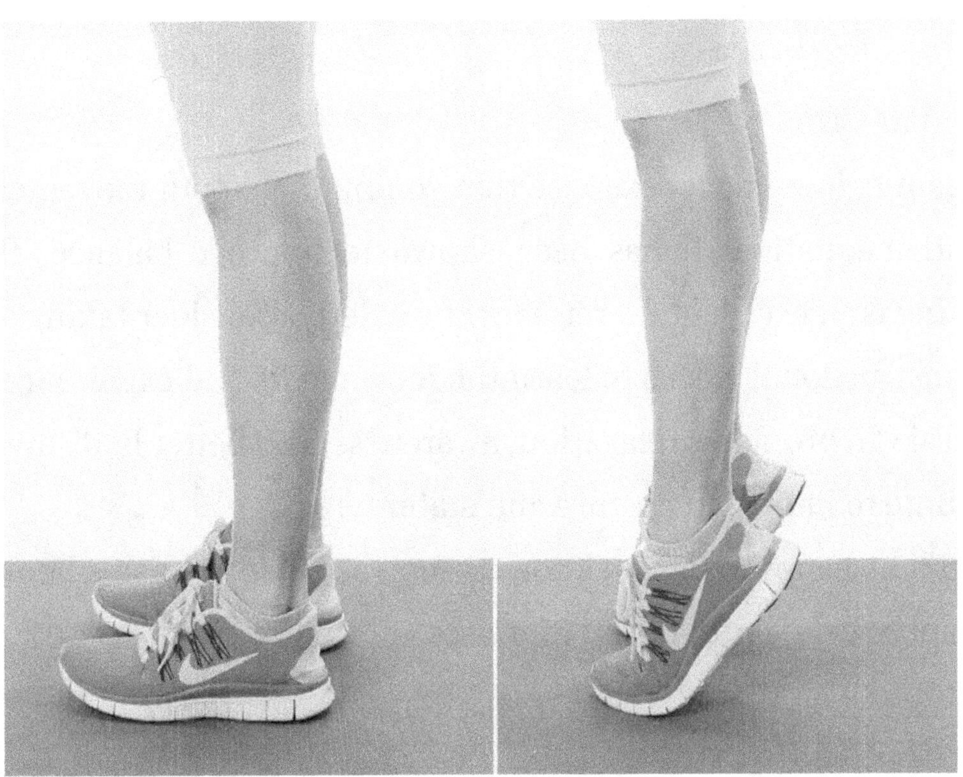

3. ARM RAISES

The arm raises exercise targets the muscles in your shoulders and upper back, helping to improve your posture and overall balance. To perform this exercise:

- Stand up straight with your feet hip-width apart and your arms resting by your sides.

- Slowly raise both arms out to the sides, keeping them straight and parallel to the ground.

- Pause for a moment, then lower your arms back down to the starting position.

- Repeat this exercise for 10-15 repetitions.

Important: Focus on maintaining proper form and avoid shrugging your shoulders or hunching forward while performing this exercise.

Remember, it's important to listen to your body and only perform exercises that are safe and comfortable for you. If you experience any pain or discomfort while performing these exercises, please consult with your healthcare provider. Stay committed to your daily exercise routine, and you'll soon reap the benefits of improved balance, posture, and confidence!

3. PRACTICE TAI CHI

Tai Chi is a gentle, low-impact exercise that combines smooth movements with deep breathing and meditation. It has been shown to improve balance, flexibility and posture, making it an excellent exercise for the elderly. Consider taking a Tai Chi class or following instructional videos to learn the movements and experience the benefits. Remember: Tai Chi promotes relaxation, awareness, and better body awareness, all of which contribute to improved posture and stability.

If you'd like, I'll be happy to let you know as soon as I also publish a book dedicated to those who want to get fit with tai chi exercises

4. STRETCH REGULARLY

Flexibility is essential for maintaining good posture and preventing muscle imbalances. Incorporate regular stretching into your daily routine to improve your range of motion and reduce muscle tension. Focus on stretching the muscles in your chest, shoulders, hips, and legs. Hold each stretch for 15-30 seconds and repeat 2-3 times on each side.

Important: Stretching helps maintain muscle balance, which is crucial for proper posture and stability.

5. USE ASSISTIVE DEVICES

If you struggle with balance or have difficulty maintaining proper posture, consider using assistive devices. These can include walking canes, walking poles, or even balance boards. Consult with a physical therapist or healthcare professional to determine which assistive device is suitable for your needs and how to use it safely. Remember: Assistive devices can provide additional support and stability, reducing the risk of falls and improving posture.

By implementing these techniques into your daily routine, you can enhance your posture and stability, ultimately improving your balance and reducing the risk of falls. Remember to start slowly and listen to your body. With consistent practice, you'll notice significant improvements in your overall well-being and confidence.

• INCORPORATING BALANCE CHALLENGES INTO DAILY ACTIVITIES

As we age, maintaining balance becomes increasingly important for our overall health and well-being. In this chapter, we will explore how to incorporate balance challenges into our daily activities, making it easier to improve our stability and prevent falls.

1. Walking: Walking is a simple yet effective way to improve balance. Try incorporating the following balance challenges into your daily walks:

- Walk on different surfaces: Vary your walking surfaces by including grass, gravel, or sand. This will engage different muscles and improve your balance.
- Walk heel-to-toe: Practice walking in a straight line, placing your heel in front of your toe with each step. This helps improve your balance and coordination.
- Walk with your eyes closed: Once you feel comfortable, try walking a short distance with your eyes closed. This challenge forces your body to rely solely on your balance and proprioception.

2. Standing: Incorporating balance challenges while standing can help strengthen your core muscles and improve your overall stability. Try the following exercises:

- Single-leg stand: Stand near a wall or countertop for support and lift one leg off the ground. Hold this position for 10-15 seconds, then switch legs. As you progress, try extending the duration of each leg lift.

- Tandem stand: Stand with one foot directly in front of the other, heel to toe. Hold this position for 10-15 seconds, then switch the position of your feet. This exercise improves your balance and coordination.
- Balance board exercises: Incorporate a balance board into your standing routine. Start by simply standing on the board and gradually progress to performing exercises like squats or lunges on the board.

3. Sitting: Even when sitting, you can still challenge your balance and improve your stability. Try these exercises:

- Marching in place: While seated, lift one foot off the ground and march in place. Focus on maintaining good posture and engaging your core muscles. Alternate between each leg for 30 seconds to 1 minute.
- Toe taps: Sit on the edge of a chair and tap your toes on the ground in a controlled manner. This exercise helps improve ankle stability and balance.
- Seated leg lifts: While seated, extend one leg straight out in front of you and hold for a few seconds. Lower your leg back down and repeat with the other leg. This exercise strengthens your leg muscles and improves balance.

4. Household activities: Many everyday activities can be turned into balance challenges. Consider the following:

- Standing on one leg while brushing your teeth or washing dishes
- Performing squats while picking up items from the floor
- Using a stability ball as a chair while working at a desk or watching TV

5. Group exercise classes: Joining a group exercise class specifically designed for seniors can be a great way to incorporate balance challenges into your routine. Look for classes that focus on activities like tai chi, yoga, or water aerobics. These classes not only improve balance but also provide a social and supportive environment.

Remember, incorporating balance challenges into your daily activities doesn't have to be complicated or time-consuming. By making small adjustments and being mindful of your movements, you can gradually improve your balance, posture, and overall confidence.

CHAPTER 5: WALKING WITH CONFIDENCE

Walking is a fundamental activity that most of us take for granted. We do it every day without much thought, relying on our balance and coordination to keep us on our feet and moving forward. But for the elderly, walking can become a source of anxiety and fear. The risk of falling and injury looms large, making every step a potential danger.

In this chapter we will explore the importance of walking for the elderly and how to do it safely. We will discuss the benefits of walking, address common concerns, and provide practical tips to help you walk with confidence and ease.

You will find practical and very easy exercises, some you already know since you have seen them in previous chapters, while others will be new and always within your reach.

THE BENEFITS OF WALKING

Walking is a low-impact exercise that offers numerous benefits for seniors. It is a weight-bearing activity that helps maintain bone density and muscle strength, reducing the risk of osteoporosis and falls. Regular walking can also improve cardiovascular health, lower blood pressure, and increase overall endurance.

Walking is not just beneficial for physical health; it also has positive effects on mental well-being. It can reduce stress, improve mood, and enhance cognitive function. Walking outdoors provides an opportunity to connect with nature, enjoy fresh air, and socialize with others.

ADDRESSING CONCERNS

Despite the many benefits, some seniors may have concerns about walking. Fear of falling is a common worry, especially if you have experienced a fall in the past. It's important to acknowledge these concerns and take steps to address them.

One way to alleviate fear is by wearing appropriate footwear. Choose shoes with good traction and support to reduce the risk of slipping or tripping. If you require additional stability, consider using a walking aid such as a cane or walker.

Another concern is walking on uneven surfaces or in unfamiliar environments. Take the time to scout your walking route beforehand, looking out for potential hazards like cracks in the pavement or uneven terrain. If necessary, walk with a companion who can provide assistance and support.

TIPS FOR WALKING WITH CONFIDENCE

Now that we have addressed some common concerns, let's explore practical tips to help you walk with confidence:

1. Start Slow and Gradually Increase Intensity: If you are new to walking or haven't been active for a while, start with short, leisurely walks. Gradually increase the duration and intensity of your walks as your fitness improves.

2. Maintain Good Posture: Stand tall, keep your head up, and look straight ahead while walking. Engage your core muscles to support your spine and maintain a stable posture.

3. Take Small Steps: Shorter steps can help improve balance and stability. Avoid overstriding, as it can throw off your balance and increase the risk of tripping.

4. Use Proper Walking Technique: Roll your foot from heel to toe with each step. This promotes a smooth, natural gait and reduces the risk of stumbling. Swing your arms naturally to maintain balance and rhythm.

5. Be Mindful of Your Surroundings: Stay alert and aware of your surroundings while walking. Look out for obstacles, uneven surfaces, or potential hazards. If you need to use a smartphone or listen to music, consider using earphones with one earpiece to maintain situational awareness.

6. Take Breaks as Needed: Listen to your body and take breaks when necessary. If you feel fatigued or lightheaded, find a safe place to rest and recover before continuing your walk.

7. Stay Hydrated: Bring a bottle of water with you and stay hydrated, especially during hot weather or longer walks. Dehydration can affect your energy levels and overall well-being.

8. Walk with a Buddy: Walking with a friend or family member not only provides companionship but also adds an extra layer of safety and support. You can motivate each other and enjoy the benefits of social interaction.

9. Practice Balance Exercises: Incorporate balance exercises into your routine to improve stability and reduce the risk of falls. Simple exercises like standing on one leg or walking heel-to-toe can help strengthen your balance muscles.

10. Stay Consistent: Make walking a regular part of your daily routine. Aim for at least 30 minutes of moderate-intensity walking most days of the week. Consistency is key to reaping the long-term benefits of walking.

By following these tips and gradually building your walking routine, you can regain confidence in your ability to walk safely and independently. Remember, every step you take is a step towards better health and a more active lifestyle.

• WALKING EXERCISES TO ENHANCE BALANCE AND COORDINATION

In this chapter, we will explore a series of walking exercises specifically designed to improve balance and coordination. Walking is a fundamental activity that we engage in every day, and by incorporating these exercises into your routine, you can enhance your stability and confidence.

EXERCISE 1: SIDE STEP WITH CROSS

This exercise targets your lateral stability and coordination. It helps improve your ability to move sideways while maintaining balance. Follow these steps to perform the side step with cross:

- Stand with your feet hip-width apart and your arms relaxed at your sides.
- Take a step to the right with your right foot, crossing it in front of your left foot.

- Step your left foot out to the left, returning to the starting position.

- Repeat the side step with cross to the right for about 10-15 steps.

- Switch directions and perform the side step with cross to the left for an equal number of steps.

Important: Maintain a slow and controlled pace throughout the exercise. Keep your knees slightly bent and your core engaged for optimal balance.

EXERCISE 2: BACKWARD WALKING

This exercise challenges your balance and coordination by reversing the direction of your steps. Here's how to perform backward walking:

- Find a clear, unobstructed path or hallway.

- Stand up straight with your feet hip-width apart.

- Turn your body to face the opposite direction.

- Take a step backward with your right foot, followed by your left foot.

- Continue walking backward for about 10-15 steps.

- If you feel unsteady, you can lightly touch a wall or countertop for support.

Important: Take small, controlled steps while walking backward. Keep your gaze forward and engage your core muscles to maintain stability.

EXERCISE 3: TANDEM WALK (SIMILAR HEEL-TO-TOE WALK)

The tandem walk exercise challenges your balance and coordination by narrowing your base of support. Here's how to perform the tandem walk:

- Find a clear, unobstructed path or hallway.

- Stand up straight with your feet together.

- Place the heel of your right foot directly in front of the toes of your left foot.

- Take a step forward with your left foot, placing the heel of your left foot directly in front of the toes of your right foot.

- Continue this heel-to-toe pattern, walking in a straight line for about 10-15 steps.

- If you feel unsteady, you can lightly touch a wall or countertop for support.

- Repeat the exercise, starting with your left foot leading.

Important: Focus on maintaining a slow and controlled pace throughout the exercise. Keep your gaze forward and engage your core muscles for added stability.

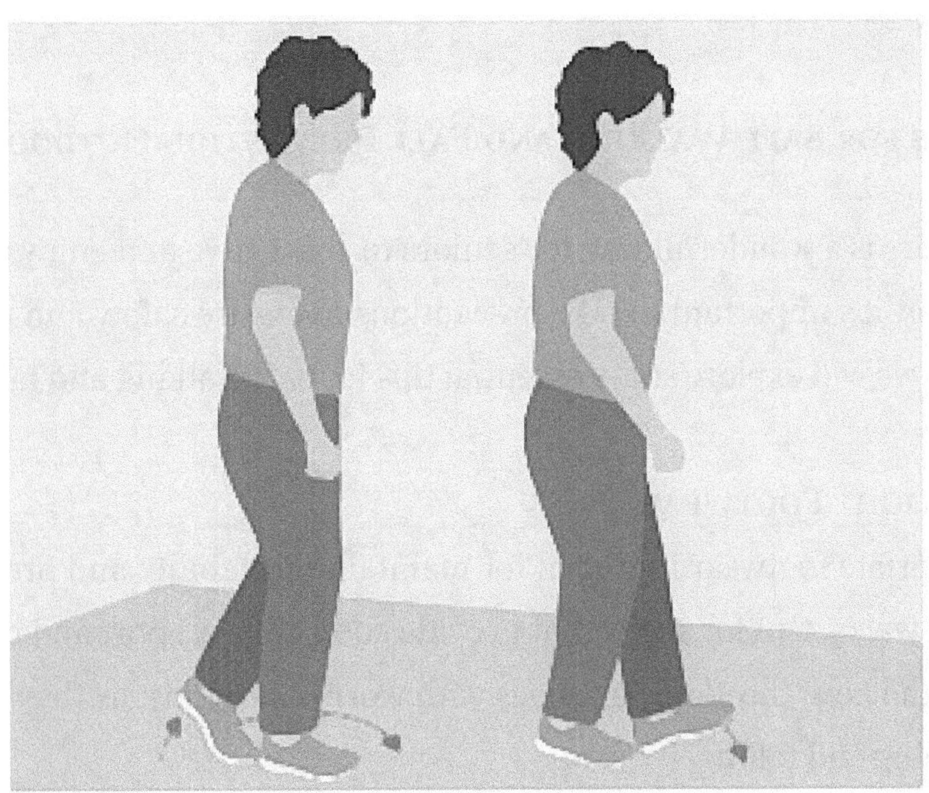

EXERCISE 3: TOE WALKING

This exercise targets the muscles in your feet and calves, which play a crucial role in balance. Follow these steps to perform toe walking:

- Stand up straight with your feet hip-width apart.

- Raise your heels off the ground, shifting your weight onto the balls of your feet.

- Walk forward on your toes for about 10-15 steps.

- If you feel unsteady, you can lightly touch a wall or countertop for support.

Important: Maintain a slow and controlled pace while walking on your toes. Keep your gaze forward and engage your core muscles for added stability.

By incorporating these walking exercises into your daily routine, you can enhance your balance, coordination, and overall stability. Remember to start slowly and gradually increase the intensity as you become more comfortable. With just five minutes a day, you can make significant improvements in your balance, posture, and confidence.

• TIPS FOR SAFE WALKING AND FALL PREVENTION OUTDOORS

Walking outdoors is a wonderful way for seniors to stay active and enjoy the beauty of nature. However, it's important to take precautions to ensure safety and prevent falls. In this chapter, we will explore some essential tips for safe walking and fall prevention outdoors.

CHOOSE THE RIGHT FOOTWEAR

Wearing appropriate footwear is crucial for maintaining stability and preventing falls during outdoor walks. Opt for shoes that provide good arch support and have non-slip soles. Avoid high heels, flip-flops, or shoes with worn-out treads, as they can increase the risk of slipping and falling.

CHECK THE WEATHER CONDITIONS

Before heading out for a walk, always check the weather forecast. Rain, snow, or icy conditions can make walking surfaces slippery and hazardous. If the weather is unfavorable, consider postponing your walk or choosing an indoor alternative, such as walking in a mall or using a treadmill.

PLAN YOUR ROUTE

Plan your walking route in advance and choose paths that are well-maintained, well-lit, and free from obstacles. Avoid uneven surfaces, cracked sidewalks, and areas with poor lighting. Consider walking in parks or designated walking trails that offer a safe and pleasant environment.

USE WALKING AIDS

If you have balance issues or feel unsteady while walking, consider using walking aids such as a cane or walker. These devices provide additional support and stability, reducing the risk of falls. Make sure to use them correctly and adjust them to the appropriate height for your comfort and stability.

BE MINDFUL OF YOUR SURROUNDINGS

Stay alert and aware of your surroundings while walking outdoors. Avoid distractions such as using your phone or listening to loud music, as they can prevent you from noticing potential hazards. Keep an eye out for uneven surfaces, potholes, or obstacles on the path and take necessary precautions to avoid them.

WALK WITH A COMPANION

Walking with a companion can enhance safety and provide additional support. Consider walking with a friend, family member, or joining a local walking group. Not only will you have someone to chat with, but you'll also have assistance in case of an emergency or if you feel unsteady during the walk.

STAY HYDRATED

Drink plenty of water before, during, and after your walk to stay hydrated. Dehydration can affect your balance and overall well-being. Carry a water bottle with you or plan your route near water fountains or restrooms where you can refill.

TAKE BREAKS AS NEEDED

Listen to your body and take breaks whenever necessary. If you feel fatigued or lightheaded, find a bench or a safe spot to rest. Don't push yourself too hard, especially if you're just starting or have any underlying health conditions. Gradually increase the duration and intensity of your walks over time.

STAY VISIBLE

If you're walking during low-light conditions or at night, make sure to wear reflective clothing or accessories to enhance visibility. Use a flashlight or headlamp to illuminate your path and make yourself more visible to others, especially if you're walking near roads or areas with vehicular traffic.

By following these tips, you can enjoy the benefits of outdoor walking while minimizing the risk of falls and injuries. Remember, safety should always be a top priority, and with a little preparation and caution, you can maintain an active and independent lifestyle.

• INTERVAL TRAINING FOR ENDURANCE AND STABILITY

Interval training is a highly effective method for improving endurance and stability, especially for seniors. By alternating periods of higher intensity exercise with periods of rest or lower intensity exercise, interval training helps to challenge the cardiovascular system and build strength and stability. This chapter will guide you through a series of interval training exercises that can be done in just a few minutes a day, helping you to improve your endurance and stability.

EXERCISE 1: MARCHING IN PLACE

Marching in place is a simple yet effective exercise that can be done anywhere. It helps to improve cardiovascular endurance and strengthen the lower body.

- Stand with your feet hip-width apart and your arms relaxed at your sides.
- Lift one knee up towards your chest, then lower it back down.
- Repeat with the other knee, alternating legs in a marching motion.
- Continue marching for 30 seconds, gradually increasing your pace as you feel comfortable.
- Rest for 15 seconds, then repeat the exercise for another 30 seconds.

Important: Keep your core engaged and maintain good posture throughout the exercise. If you have difficulty balancing, you can hold onto a stable surface for support.

EXERCISE 2: STEP-UPS

Step-ups are a great exercise for building lower body strength and improving balance. You can use a step or a sturdy platform for this exercise.

- Stand in front of the step or platform with your feet hip-width apart.

- Place one foot on the step, pressing through your heel to lift your body up.

- Step back down with the same foot, returning to the starting position.

- Repeat the exercise with the other foot, alternating legs for 10 repetitions.

- Rest for 15 seconds, then complete 2 more sets of 10 repetitions, resting for 15 seconds between each set.

Important: Keep your core engaged and maintain good posture throughout the exercise. If you have difficulty balancing, you can hold onto a stable surface for support. Start with a lower step or platform height and gradually increase the height as you feel comfortable.

EXERCISE 3: HIGH KNEE MARCH

The high knee march is a dynamic exercise that helps to improve cardiovascular endurance, strengthen the lower body, and improve balance.

- Stand with your feet hip-width apart and your arms relaxed at your sides.

- Lift one knee up towards your chest as high as you can, while swinging the opposite arm forward.

- Lower your leg and arm back down, then repeat with the other leg and arm.

- Continue alternating legs for 30 seconds, gradually increasing your pace as you feel comfortable.

- Rest for 15 seconds, then repeat the exercise for another 30 seconds.

Important: Keep your core engaged and maintain good posture throughout the exercise. If you have difficulty balancing, you can hold onto a stable surface for support.

Remember, interval training can be customized to your fitness level and abilities. Start with shorter intervals and gradually increase the duration and intensity as you feel comfortable. It's always important to listen to your body and modify exercises as needed. By incorporating these interval training exercises into your daily routine, you can improve your endurance and stability, helping you to maintain an active and independent lifestyle.

Chapter 6: Core Strength and Stability

Welcome back, my dear readers! Today, we dive into the world of core strength and stability. Our core muscles are the foundation of our bodies, providing support and balance in everything we do. As we age, it becomes even more crucial to strengthen these muscles to maintain our independence and prevent falls. So, let's get started on our journey to a stronger and more stable core!

Why is Core Strength Important?

Our core muscles, which include the abdominals, back muscles, and pelvic floor, play a vital role in maintaining our balance and stability. They provide support to our spine, pelvis, and hips, allowing us to perform everyday activities with ease and confidence. As we age, our core muscles tend to weaken, leading to poor posture, decreased stability, and an increased risk of falls. By strengthening our core, we can improve our balance, posture, and overall well-being. So, let's not wait any longer and start incorporating some simple yet effective exercises into our daily routine!

• Techniques to Enhance Posture and Stability

Good posture and stability are essential for maintaining balance and preventing falls, especially for seniors. In this chapter, we will explore various techniques that can help enhance your posture and stability, ultimately improving your overall balance and confidence.

1. ALIGN YOUR SPINE

Proper alignment of the spine is crucial for maintaining good posture. Start by standing with your feet hip-width apart and your shoulders relaxed. Imagine a straight line extending from the top of your head down to your tailbone. Engage your core muscles to support your spine and avoid slouching. Practice this alignment throughout the day, whether you're sitting, standing, or walking.

Remember: A straight spine promotes better balance and reduces strain on your joints.

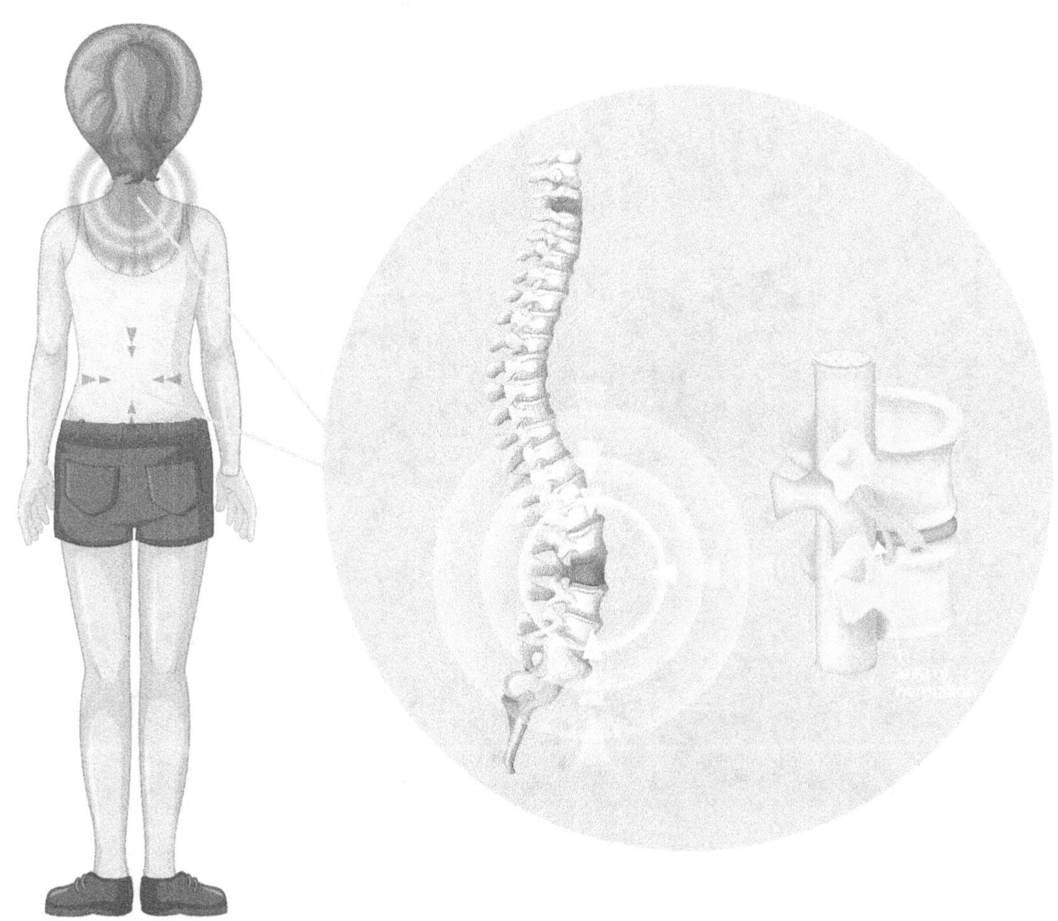

2. STRENGTHENING THE CORE

Core muscles play an important role in maintaining stability and balance. To strengthen the core, you need to perform targeted exercises for the abdominal and back muscles. Some effective exercises are:

- <u>Bridge</u>: Lie on your back with your knees bent and your feet resting on the floor. Lift your hips off the floor, creating a straight line from your knees to your shoulders. Hold this position for 10-15 seconds, then lower the hips again. Repeat 8-10 times.

- <u>Superman</u>: Lie face down on the floor with your arms stretched out in front of you. Simultaneously raise your arms, chest and legs off the floor, engaging your core muscles. Hold the position for a few seconds, then lower yourself. Repeat 4-6 times. Important: Strong core muscles provide stability and support to the whole body, improving balance and posture.

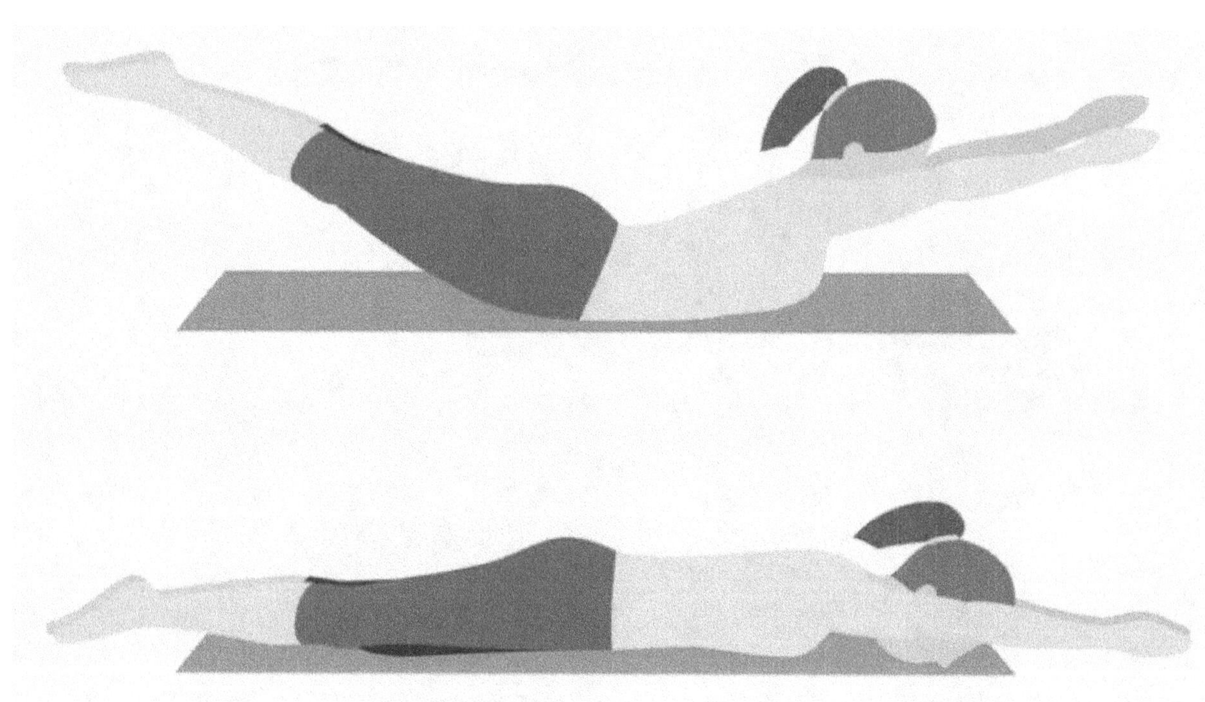

EXERCISE 3: PLANK

The plank is a highly effective exercise for strengthening your core muscles. To perform the plank:

- Start by positioning yourself face down on the floor, resting on your forearms and toes.
- Engage your abdominal muscles and lift your body off the floor, maintaining a straight line from your head to your heels.

- Hold this position for 20 seconds, focusing on keeping your core muscles engaged.
- Slowly lower your body back down to the starting position.

Important: Make sure to keep your back straight and avoid sagging or arching your lower back during the exercise. If you find it challenging to maintain the full plank position, you can modify it by resting on your knees instead of your toes.

EXERCISE 4: STANDING SIDE LEG LIFTS

Standing side leg lifts are an effective exercise for improving balance and stability in your hips and legs. To perform standing side leg lifts:

- Stand tall with your feet hip-width apart and your hands resting on a sturdy surface for support.
- Shift your weight onto your left leg and lift your right leg out to the side, keeping it straight.
- Hold this position for 15-20 seconds, focusing on maintaining your balance.
- Lower your right leg back down and repeat on the opposite side.

Important: Keep your core muscles engaged throughout the exercise to help improve your stability. If needed, you can perform this exercise while holding onto a chair or countertop for additional support.

EXERCISE 5: BIRD DOG

The bird dog exercise is excellent for improving balance and stability by targeting the muscles in your back and abdomen. To perform the bird dog:

- Start on your hands and knees, with your hands directly under your shoulders and your knees under your hips.
- Extend your right arm forward while simultaneously extending your left leg backward.
- Hold this position for 20 seconds, focusing on keeping your core muscles engaged.

- Return to the starting position and repeat on the opposite side.

Important: Be mindful of maintaining a neutral spine throughout the exercise, avoiding any excessive arching or rounding of your back. Keep your movements slow and controlled, focusing on balance and stability.

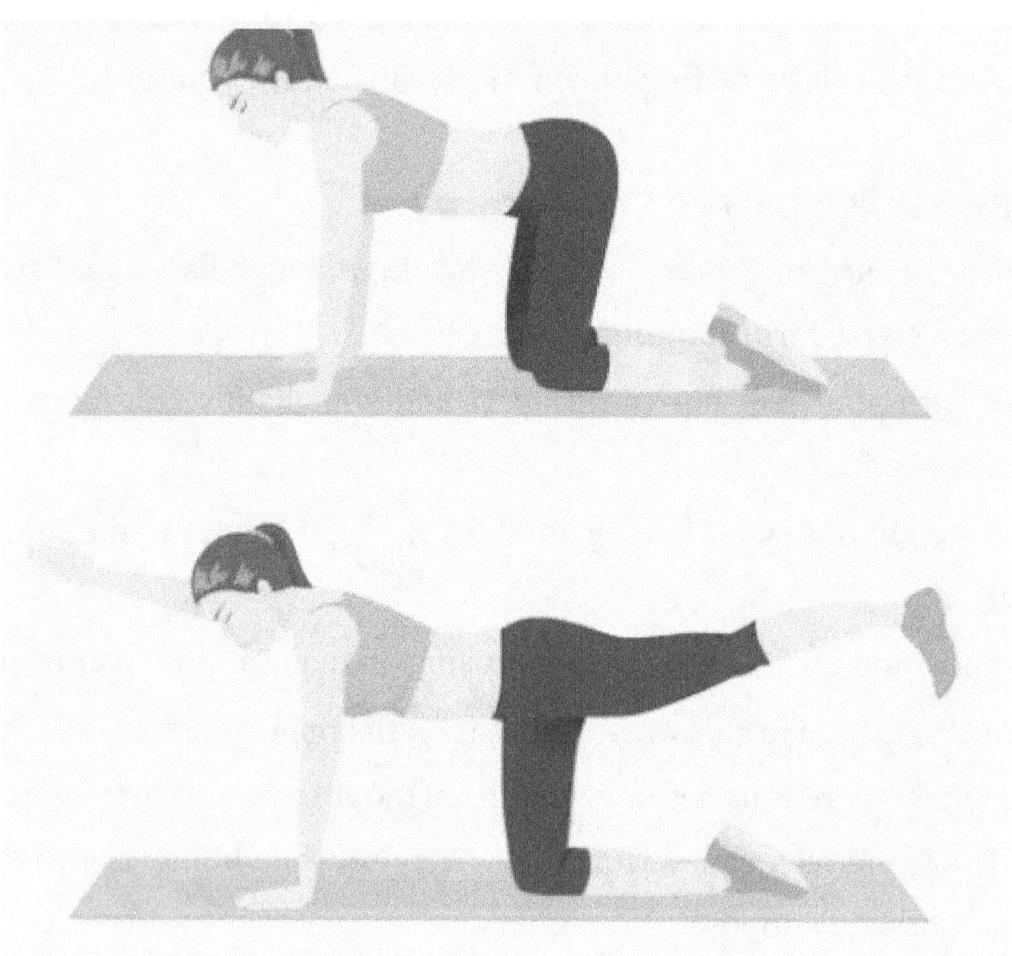

EXERCISE 6: WALL PUSH-UPS

Wall push-ups are a modified version of traditional push-ups that can be done against a wall. They help to strengthen the upper body and improve stability.

- Stand facing a wall, about arm's length away.
- Place your hands on the wall at shoulder height, slightly wider than shoulder-width apart.
- Step back a few feet, keeping your body straight and your feet hip-width apart.
- Bend your elbows and lower your chest towards the wall, keeping your back straight.

- Push yourself back up to the starting position.

- Repeat the exercise for 10 repetitions, then rest for 15 seconds.

- Complete 2 more sets of 10 repetitions, resting for 15 seconds between each set.

Important: Make sure to maintain proper form throughout the exercise. Keep your core engaged and avoid arching your back. If you have shoulder or wrist pain, you can modify the exercise by performing it against a sturdy countertop or table instead of a wall.

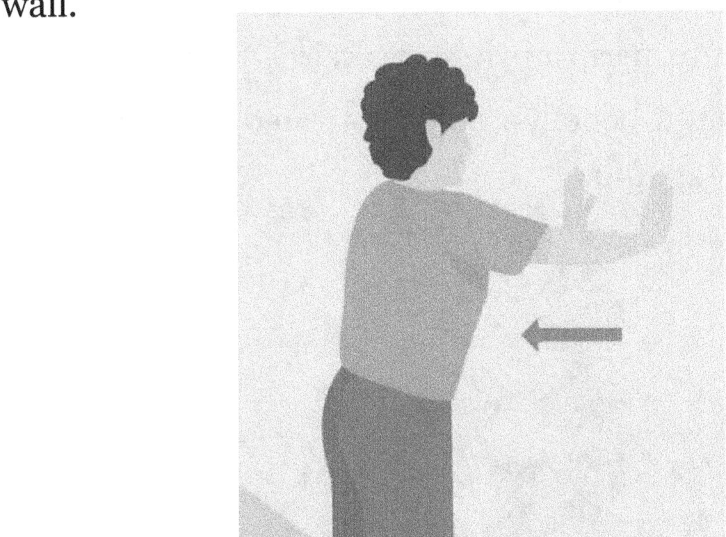
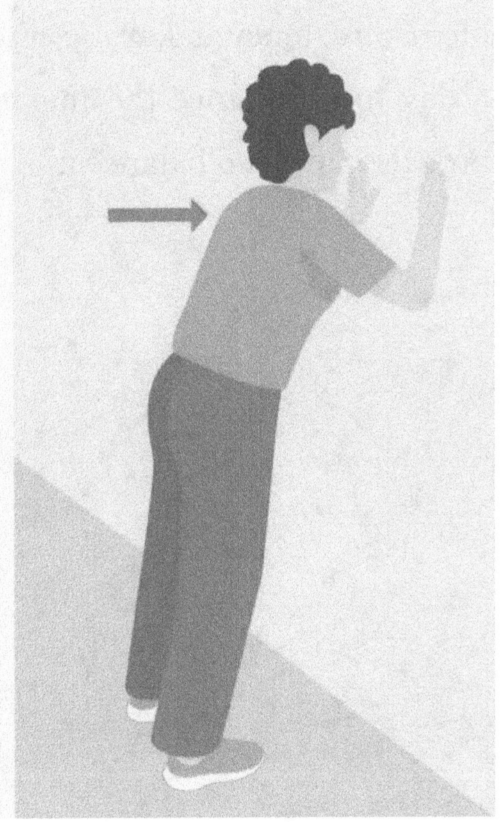

EXERCISE 7: SEATED RUSSIAN TWISTS

Seated Russian twists are a seated exercise that targets your oblique muscles, helping to improve rotational stability. To perform seated Russian twists:

- Sit on the edge of a sturdy chair or bench, with your feet flat on the floor and your knees bent.

- Lean back slightly, engaging your core muscles.

- Twist your torso to the right, bringing your left hand towards your right hip.

- Return to the center and repeat on the opposite side.

Important: Avoid straining your neck or back during this exercise. Keep your movements controlled and focus on engaging your core muscles throughout the twisting motion.

By incorporating these core exercises into your daily routine, you can enhance your balance, stability, and overall posture. Remember to start gradually and listen to your body, gradually increasing the duration or intensity of the exercises as you feel comfortable. Consistency is key, so aim to perform these exercises for at least five minutes a day to experience the maximum benefits. Stay motivated and enjoy the journey towards improved balance and stability!

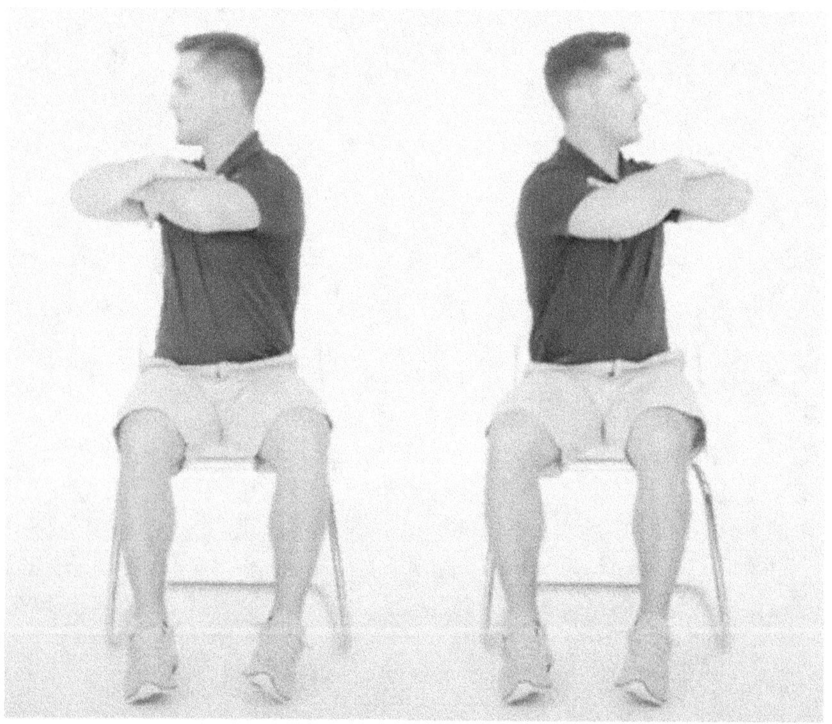

CORE STRENGTHENING WORKOUTS

Welcome to the Core Strengthening Workouts chapter! In this section, we will focus on exercises that target your core muscles, which are essential for maintaining balance and stability. By strengthening your core, you will improve your posture, reduce the risk of falls, and enhance your overall physical well-being. These exercises can be easily incorporated into your daily routine, and with just a few minutes a day, you can make significant progress. Let's get started!

EXERCISE 1: SEATED LEG LIFTS

This exercise is designed to strengthen your abdominal muscles and hip flexors.

Instructions:

- Sit on a sturdy chair with your feet flat on the floor and your back straight.
- Slowly lift one leg straight out in front of you, keeping your knee straight.
- Hold for a few seconds, then lower your leg back down.
- Repeat with the other leg.

Important: Engage your core muscles throughout the exercise and avoid leaning or using your arms for support.

EXERCISE 2: BRIDGE

The bridge exercise targets your glutes, hamstrings, and lower back muscles, helping to improve core stability.

Instructions:

- Lie on your back with your knees bent and your feet flat on the floor.
- Place your hands by your sides, palms down.
- Engage your core muscles and lift your hips off the floor, forming a straight line from your knees to your shoulders.
- Hold this position for a few seconds, then slowly lower your hips back down.

Important: Avoid arching your back or pushing your hips too high. Focus on using your glutes and hamstrings to lift your hips.

EXERCISE 4: STANDING SIDE CRUNCHES

This exercise targets your oblique muscles, which are essential for maintaining balance and stability.

Instructions:

- Stand with your feet shoulder-width apart and your arms by your sides.
- Place your right hand on your right hip and extend your left arm overhead.
- Engage your core muscles and bend sideways to the right, squeezing your oblique muscles.
- Return to the starting position and repeat on the other side.

Important: Keep your movements controlled and avoid leaning forward or backward. Focus on using your core muscles to initiate the movement.

EXERCISE 5: SILVER SURFER

This exercise targets the lower back muscles, which play a key role in maintaining good posture.

Instructions:

- Lie on your stomach with your arms extended along your sides and legs straight.

- Engage your core muscles and simultaneously lift your arms and legs off the floor.

- Hold this position for a few seconds, then lower your arms and legs back down.

Important: Avoid straining the neck or back. Focus on using your lower back muscles to lift your upper body and legs.

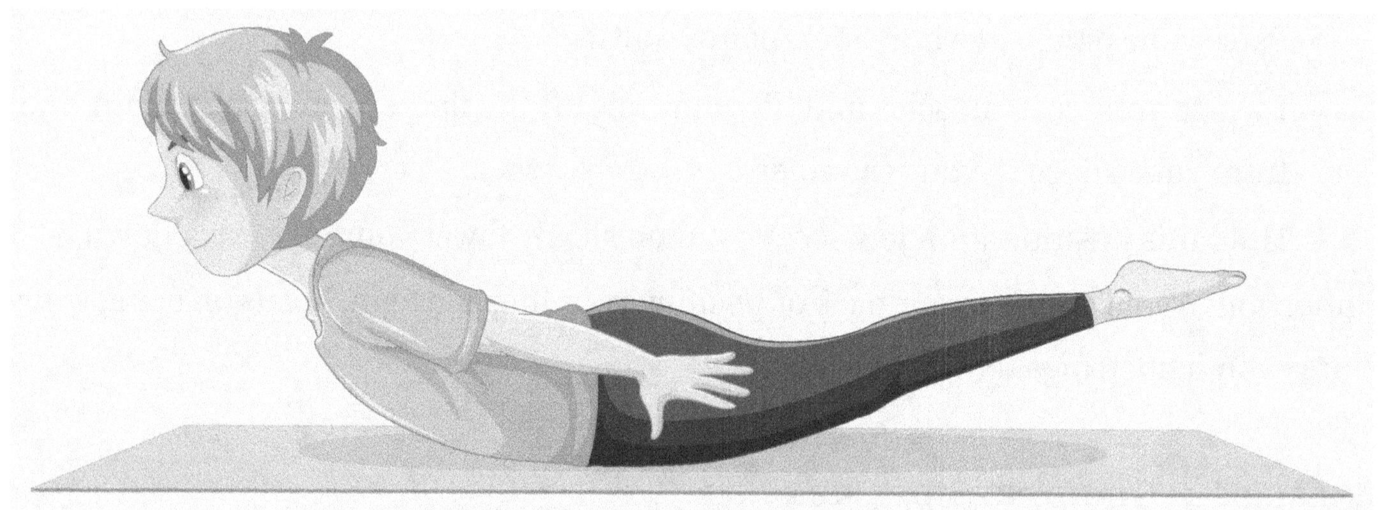

EXERCISE 2: FULL PLANK

The plank is a classic exercise that targets your entire core, including your abdominals, back muscles, and glutes.

Instructions:

- Start by getting into a push-up position, with your hands directly under your shoulders and your toes on the floor.
- Engage your core muscles and maintain a straight line from your head to your heels.
- Hold this position for as long as you can, aiming for at least 30 seconds.
- Remember to breathe evenly throughout the exercise.

Important: If the full plank position is too challenging, you can modify it by resting on your forearms instead of your hands.

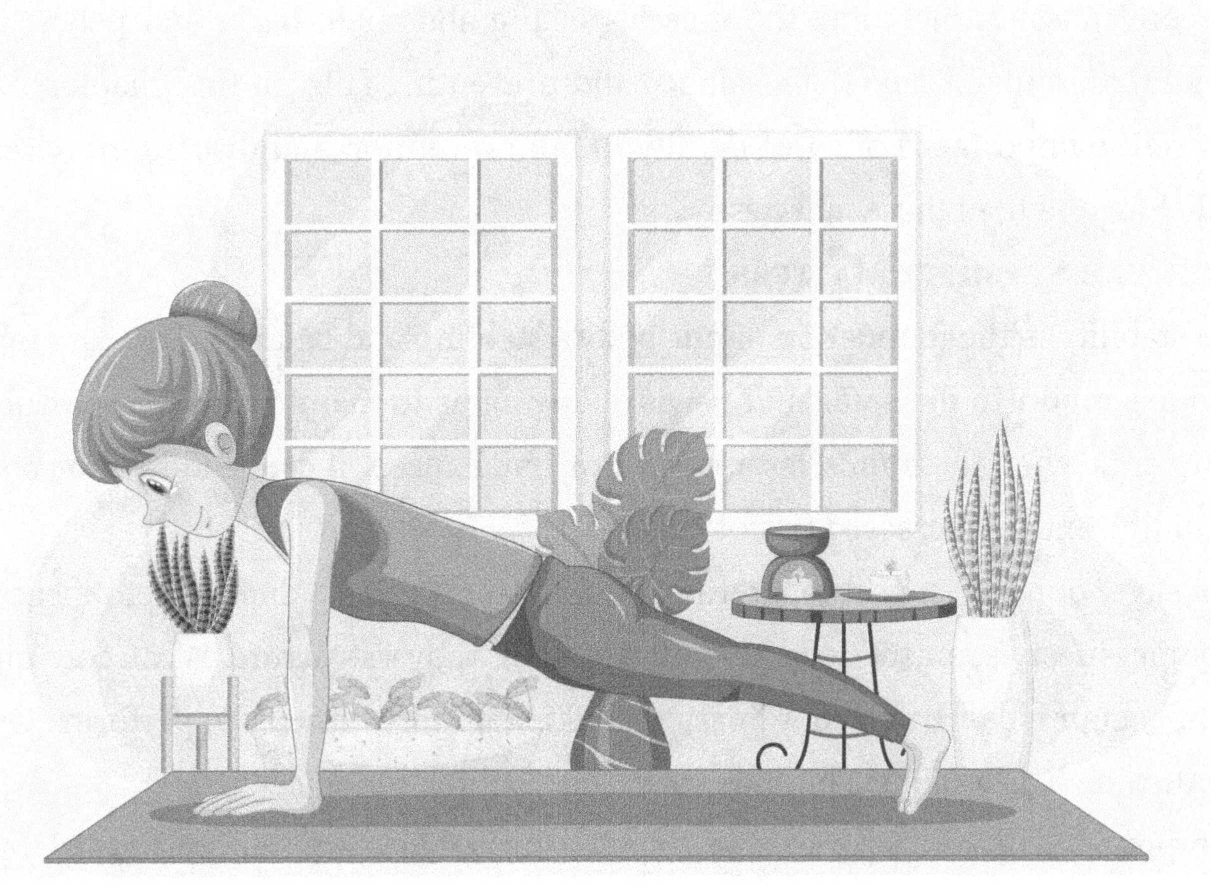

Congratulations on completing the Core Strengthening Workouts chapter! By incorporating these exercises into your daily routine, you are taking important steps towards improving your balance, posture, and overall well-being. Remember to start slowly and gradually increase the intensity and duration of your workouts. Stay motivated and consistent, and you will soon experience the benefits of a stronger core. In the next chapter, we will explore exercises that target your lower body muscles. Keep up the great work!

• IMPORTANCE OF CORE STABILITY IN FALL PREVENTION

As we age, maintaining balance becomes increasingly important for preventing falls and maintaining our independence. One key component of balance is core stability. The core muscles, including the muscles of the abdomen, back, and pelvis, play a crucial role in maintaining our balance and preventing falls. In this chapter, we will explore the importance of core stability in fall prevention and discuss exercises that can help strengthen these muscles.

WHY CORE STABILITY MATTERS

Core stability is the foundation of our body's stability and balance. The core muscles provide support to the spine and pelvis, allowing us to maintain proper posture and alignment. When these muscles are weak or imbalanced, it can lead to poor posture, instability, and an increased risk of falls.

As we age, our core muscles naturally weaken. This can be due to factors such as a sedentary lifestyle, muscle loss, or changes in our body's structure. Weak core muscles can affect our balance and coordination, making it more difficult to perform everyday activities such as walking, climbing stairs, or reaching for objects.

By improving core stability, we can enhance our balance and reduce the risk of falls. Strong core muscles provide a solid foundation for our body, allowing us to maintain proper alignment and control our movements. When our core is stable, we are less likely to lose our balance or experience sudden shifts in weight distribution that can lead to falls.

EXERCISES TO IMPROVE CORE STABILITY

Here are some simple exercises that can help strengthen your core muscles:

- Leg Raises: Lie on your back with your legs extended and your arms at your sides. Engage your core muscles and lift one leg off the floor, keeping it straight. Hold for a few seconds, then lower your leg back down. Repeat on the other side. Aim for 10-12 repetitions on each leg.
- Standing Side Leg Lifts: Stand behind a sturdy chair, holding onto the back for support. Engage your core muscles and lift one leg out to the side, keeping it straight. Hold for a few seconds, then lower your leg back down. Repeat on the other side. Aim for 10-12 repetitions on each leg.

Remember to breathe deeply and maintain proper form throughout each exercise. If you have any existing health conditions or concerns, it's always a good idea to consult with your healthcare provider before starting a new exercise program.

Core stability is essential for maintaining balance and preventing falls as we age. By incorporating exercises that target the core muscles into our daily routine, we can improve our balance, posture, and overall well-being. Remember, consistency is key. Aim to perform these exercises for just a few minutes each day, and over time, you'll notice a significant improvement in your core strength and stability.

Next, we will explore the role of flexibility in fall prevention and discuss exercises that can help improve our range of motion and mobility. Stay tuned!

Chapter 7: Vestibular Exercises

In this chapter, we will explore a series of exercises that specifically target the vestibular system, which plays a crucial role in maintaining our balance and spatial orientation. These exercises will help improve your body's ability to sense and respond to changes in position and movement, ultimately enhancing your overall stability and reducing the risk of falls.

The Importance of the Vestibular System

Before we dive into the exercises, let's take a moment to understand the significance of the vestibular system. Located within the inner ear, this complex network of structures and nerves is responsible for detecting changes in head position and movement. It works in tandem with our visual system and proprioception (our body's sense of where it is in space) to help us maintain our balance and coordinate our movements.

Think of the vestibular system as your body's internal GPS, constantly providing feedback about your position and movement in relation to your surroundings.

Exercise 1: Head Turns

Head turns are a simple yet effective way to stimulate the vestibular system and improve its function. To perform this exercise:

- Sit or stand in a comfortable position with your feet shoulder-width apart.
- Gently turn your head to the right as far as you can without straining.
- Hold this position for a few seconds, then slowly return your head to the center.
- Repeat the movement, this time turning your head to the left.
- Continue alternating between right and left head turns for 1 minute.

Remember to move your head slowly and smoothly, without jerking or forcing the movement.

EXERCISE 2: EYE TRACKING

Eye tracking exercises help improve the coordination between your vestibular and visual systems. To perform this exercise:

- Find a small object or spot on the wall at eye level.
- Focus your gaze on the object and keep your head still.
- Slowly move your eyes from side to side, tracking the object with your gaze.
- After a few seconds, change the direction of your eye movements, tracking the object up and down.
- Continue alternating between horizontal and vertical eye movements for 1 minute.

Make sure to move your eyes smoothly and without straining.

EXERCISE 3: TANDEM WALKING

Tandem walking is a challenging exercise that helps improve your balance and coordination by narrowing your base of support. To perform this exercise:

- Find a clear space where you have enough room to take several steps forward.
- Stand with one foot directly in front of the other, placing your heel against the toes of the opposite foot.
- Keep your arms relaxed by your sides and your gaze focused straight ahead.
- Take slow, deliberate steps forward, placing one foot directly in front of the other.
- Continue walking in this manner for 1 minute.

Take your time and maintain a steady pace as you perform tandem walking. If you feel unsteady, you can lightly touch a wall or piece of furniture for support.

EXERCISE 4: TAI CHI "CLOUD" BALANCE EXERCISE

Tai Chi is a gentle, flowing martial art that has been shown to improve balance and reduce the risk of falls in older adults. The following exercise is a simplified version of a Tai Chi movement called "Cloud Hands." To perform this exercise:

- Stand with your feet shoulder-width apart and your knees slightly bent.
- Extend your arms in front of you, palms facing down.
- Shift your weight to your left foot and pivot on your right foot, turning your body to the right.
- As you turn, let your arms follow the movement, sweeping them to the right.
- Shift your weight back to your right foot and pivot on your left foot, turning your body to the left.
- Again, let your arms follow the movement, sweeping them to the left.
- Continue shifting your weight and pivoting from side to side for 1 minute.

Focus on maintaining a smooth, continuous flow of movement as you perform this exercise.

EXERCISE 5: STANDING BALANCE WITH HEAD TURNS

This exercise combines head turns with standing balance to ch your vestibular system further. To perform this exercise:

- Stand with your feet hip-width apart and your arms relaxed by your sides.
- Gently turn your head to the right as far as you can without losing your balance.
- Hold this position for a few seconds, then slowly return your head to the center.
- Repeat the movement, this time turning your head to the left.
- Continue alternating between right and left head turns while maintaining your balance for 1 minute.

Remember to engage your core muscles and focus on a fixed point in front of you to help maintain your balance.

By incorporating these vestibular exercises into your daily routine, you can strengthen your balance, improve your posture, and enhance your overall confidence. Remember, consistency is key, so aim to perform these exercises for at least five minutes each day. With time and practice, you'll notice a significant improvement in your stability and well-being.

• **TECHNIQUES TO IMPROVE VESTIBULAR FUNCTION AND BALANCE**

From here on, I will explain the exercises by listing the following lineup of information each time, which is useful to be even clearer about the functionality of the exercise you are practicing.

Lineup of information:
Exercise:
Objective of the exercise:
Level of difficulty:
Equipment needed:
Detailed description:
Key points:
Benefits:
Variations and adaptations:
Frequency and duration:

Some of the exercises you will find below you already know but don't worry. In this chapter you will have to perform them as best you can and with the experience of past chapters. Are you ready? Let's get started!

<u>Exercise 1: Standing Heel-to-Toe</u>

Objective of the Exercise: To improve balance and coordination by challenging the vestibular system.

Difficulty Level: Beginner

Equipment Needed: A sturdy chair or countertop for support.

Detailed Description:

- Stand tall with your feet together, touching heel-to-toe.
- Place your hands on the back of a chair or a countertop for support.
- Focus your gaze on a fixed point in front of you.
- Take slow, deliberate steps forward, placing one foot directly in front of the other.
- Continue walking heel-to-toe for a few steps, maintaining your balance.
- Turn around and repeat the exercise in the opposite direction.

Key Focus Points:

- Engage your core muscles to help maintain stability.
- Keep your gaze fixed on a stable point to improve focus and balance.
- Take slow, deliberate steps to challenge your balance and coordination.
- Use the chair or countertop for support if needed.

Benefits:

- Enhances balance and coordination, reducing the risk of falls.
- Strengthens the leg muscles and improves posture.
- Challenges the vestibular system, improving its function over time.

Variations and Adaptations:

- If you feel unsteady, perform the exercise near a wall for added support.
- As you become more comfortable, try performing the exercise without holding onto anything for support.

Frequency and Duration: Perform 10 steps in each direction, twice a day.

<u>Exercise 2: Single Leg Balance</u>

Objective of the Exercise: To improve balance and strengthen the leg muscles.

Difficulty Level: Beginner

Equipment Needed: A sturdy chair or countertop for support.

Detailed Description:

- Stand tall behind a chair or countertop, holding onto it for support.
- Shift your weight onto your left leg while lifting your right foot off the ground.
- Bend your left knee slightly and engage your core muscles for stability.
- Hold this position for 10 seconds, maintaining your balance.
- Slowly lower your right foot back to the ground.
- Repeat the exercise on the opposite leg.

Key Focus Points:

- Keep your gaze fixed on a stable point to improve focus and balance.
- Engage your core muscles to help maintain stability.
- Avoid locking your standing knee; keep it slightly bent.
- Use the chair or countertop for support if needed.

Benefits:

- Improves balance and stability, reducing the risk of falls.
- Strengthens the leg muscles, particularly the quadriceps and calves.
- Enhances proprioception, the body's awareness of its position in space.

Variations and Adaptations:

- If you feel unsteady, perform the exercise near a wall for added support.
- As you become more comfortable, try performing the exercise without holding onto anything for support.

Frequency and Duration: Hold the single leg balance for 10 seconds on each leg, twice a day.

<u>Exercise 3: Standing Leg Swings</u>

Objective of the Exercise: To improve balance, hip flexibility, and leg strength.

Difficulty Level: Intermediate

Equipment Needed: A clear, unobstructed space.

Detailed Description:

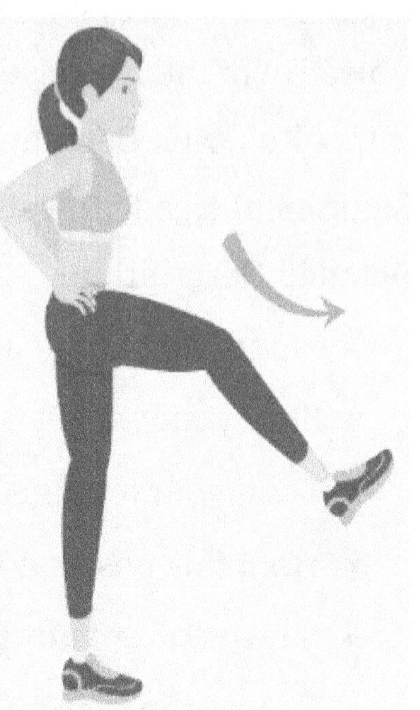

- Stand tall with your feet hip-width apart, arms relaxed at your sides.
- Shift your weight onto your left leg, keeping a slight bend in the knee.
- Swing your right leg forward and backward, maintaining your balance.
- Continue swinging your leg, gradually increasing the range of motion.
- Switch to the opposite leg and repeat the exercise.

Key Focus Points:

- Engage your core muscles to help maintain stability.
- Keep your gaze fixed on a stable point to improve focus and balance.
- Move smoothly and control the swinging motion of your leg.

Benefits:

- Improves balance, hip flexibility, and leg strength.
- Enhances coordination and proprioception.
- Increases blood flow to the legs, promoting overall lower body health.

Variations and Adaptations:

- If you feel unsteady, perform the exercise near a wall for added support.
- As you become more comfortable, try performing the exercise with your eyes closed.

Frequency and Duration: Swing each leg for 10 repetitions, twice a day.

<u>Exercise 4: Calf Raises</u>

Objective of the Exercise: To strengthen the calf muscles and improve balance.

Difficulty Level: Beginner

Equipment Needed: A sturdy chair or countertop for support.

Detailed Description:

- Stand tall behind a chair or countertop, holding onto it for support.
- Place your feet shoulder-width apart, toes pointing forward.
- Raise your heels off the ground, lifting your body onto the balls of your feet.
- Hold this position for a moment, then slowly lower your heels back to the ground.
- Repeat the exercise, focusing on maintaining your balance throughout.

Key Focus Points:

- Engage your core muscles to help maintain stability.
- Keep your gaze fixed on a stable point to improve focus and balance.
- Move smoothly and control your descent when lowering your heels.
- Use the chair or countertop for support if needed.

Benefits:

- Strengthens the calf muscles, improving lower leg strength and stability.
- Enhances ankle mobility and balance.
- Improves overall lower body strength and endurance.

Variations and Adaptations:

- If you feel unsteady, perform the exercise near a wall for added support.
- As you become more comfortable, try performing the exercise without holding onto anything for support.

Frequency and Duration: Perform 10 repetitions of calf raises, twice a day.

<u>Exercise 5: Side Leg Raises</u>

Objective of the Exercise: To strengthen the hip abductor muscles and improve balance.

Difficulty Level: Beginner

Equipment Needed: A clear, unobstructed space.

Detailed Description:

- Stand tall with your feet hip-width apart, arms relaxed at your sides.
- Shift your weight onto your left leg, keeping a slight bend in the knee.
- Raise your right leg out to the side, keeping it straight.
- Hold this position for a moment, then lower your leg back to the starting position.
- Repeat the exercise, focusing on maintaining your balance throughout.
- Switch to the opposite leg and repeat the exercise.

Key Focus Points:

- Engage your core muscles to help maintain stability.
- Keep your gaze fixed on a stable point to improve focus and balance.
- Move smoothly and control the lifting and lowering of your leg.

Benefits:

- Strengthens the hip abductor muscles, improving stability and balance.
- Enhances hip mobility and flexibility.
- Improves overall lower body strength and endurance.

Variations and Adaptations:

- If you feel unsteady, perform the exercise near a wall for added support.
- As you become more comfortable, try performing the exercise without holding onto anything for support.

Frequency and Duration: Perform 10 repetitions of side leg raises on each leg, twice a day.

Exercise 6: Standing March

Objective of the Exercise: To improve balance, coordination, and leg strength.

Difficulty Level: Beginner

Equipment Needed: A clear, unobstructed space.

Detailed Description:

- Stand tall with your feet hip-width apart, arms relaxed at your sides.
- Shift your weight onto your left leg, keeping a slight bend in the knee.
- Lift your right knee up towards your chest, while balancing on your left leg.
- Lower your right leg back down to the ground, and repeat the exercise on the opposite side.
- Continue alternating legs, marching in place.

Key Focus Points:

- Engage your core muscles to help maintain stability.
- Keep your gaze fixed on a stable point to improve focus and balance.
- Move smoothly and control the lifting and lowering of your legs.

Benefits:

- Improves balance, coordination, and leg strength.
- Enhances hip mobility and flexibility.
- Challenges the cardiovascular system, promoting overall fitness.

Variations and Adaptations:

- If you feel unsteady, perform the exercise near a wall for added support.
- As you become more comfortable, try marching in place without holding onto anything for support.

Frequency and Duration: March in place for 10 repetitions on each leg, twice a day.

• EXERCISES TO REDUCE DIZZINESS AND VERTIGO SYMPTOMS

Exercise: Heel-to-Toe Walk

Objective of the Exercise: To improve balance and coordination by practicing a heel-to-toe walking pattern.

Difficulty Level: Beginner

Equipment Needed: A clear, open space

Detailed Description:

- Stand up straight with your feet together, arms by your sides.
- Take a step forward with your right foot, placing your right heel directly in front of your left toes.
- Shift your weight onto your right foot and bring your left foot forward, placing your left heel directly in front of your right toes.
- Continue this heel-to-toe pattern, walking in a straight line.
- Keep your gaze forward and engage your core for balance.

Key Focus Points:

- Maintain a slow and controlled pace throughout the exercise.
- Focus on keeping your heel and toes in a straight line as you step.
- Try to avoid looking down at your feet; instead, keep your eyes focused on a point in front of you.
- If you feel unsteady, you can lightly touch a wall or countertop for support.

Benefits:

- Enhances balance and coordination, which can help prevent falls.
- Strengthens the muscles in the legs and core.
- Improves proprioception, the body's awareness of its position in space.

Variations and Adaptations:

- If walking in a straight line is challenging, start by practicing the heel-to-toe pattern while standing in place.
- You can also perform this exercise while holding onto a sturdy chair or countertop for added support.

Frequency and Duration: Aim to perform this exercise for 1-2 minutes, twice a day.

Exercise: Single Leg Stand

Objective of the Exercise: To improve balance and strengthen the muscles in the legs and core by standing on one leg.

Difficulty Level: Beginner

Equipment Needed: A sturdy chair or countertop for support

Detailed Description:

- Stand up straight, holding onto a sturdy chair or countertop for support.
- Lift your right foot off the ground, bending your knee slightly.
- Try to balance on your left leg for as long as you can, keeping your posture upright.
- If needed, you can lightly touch the support with your fingertips for stability.
- Repeat on the other leg.

Key Focus Points:

- Keep your gaze forward and fix your eyes on a point in front of you to help with balance.
- Engage your core muscles to help stabilize your body.
- If you feel unsteady, focus on your breath and try to relax your body.
- Start with a shorter duration and gradually increase the time as you build strength and balance.

Benefits:

- Strengthens the muscles in the legs, particularly the calves and quadriceps.
- Improves balance and stability, reducing the risk of falls.
- Enhances proprioception and body awareness.

Variations and Adaptations:

- If standing on one leg is too challenging, you can perform this exercise while holding onto a support with both hands.
- You can also practice balancing on a foam pad or pillow to increase the difficulty.

Frequency and Duration: Aim to perform this exercise for 30 seconds to 1 minute on each leg, twice a day.

<u>Exercise: Toe Taps</u>

Objective of the Exercise: To improve balance and strengthen the muscles in the lower body by tapping the toes on an elevated surface.

Difficulty Level: Beginner

Equipment Needed: A sturdy step or low platform

Detailed Description:

- Stand in front of a sturdy step or low platform.
- Lift your right foot and tap your toes on the step, then lower your foot back down to the ground.
- Repeat this movement with your left foot, tapping your toes on the step and returning to the ground.
- Continue alternating between the right and left foot, tapping the toes on the step.

Key Focus Points:

- Keep your posture upright and your gaze forward throughout the exercise.
- Engage your core muscles to help with balance and stability.
- Avoid rushing the movement; maintain a controlled and steady pace.
- If needed, lightly touch a support with your fingertips for stability.

Benefits:

- Strengthens the muscles in the legs, particularly the calves and quadriceps.
- Improves balance and stability, reducing the risk of falls.
- Enhances ankle flexibility and range of motion.

Variations and Adaptations:

- If tapping the toes on a step is too challenging, you can start by tapping the toes on the ground.
- You can also increase the difficulty by using a higher step or platform.

Frequency and Duration: Aim to perform this exercise for 10-12 repetitions on each foot, twice a day.

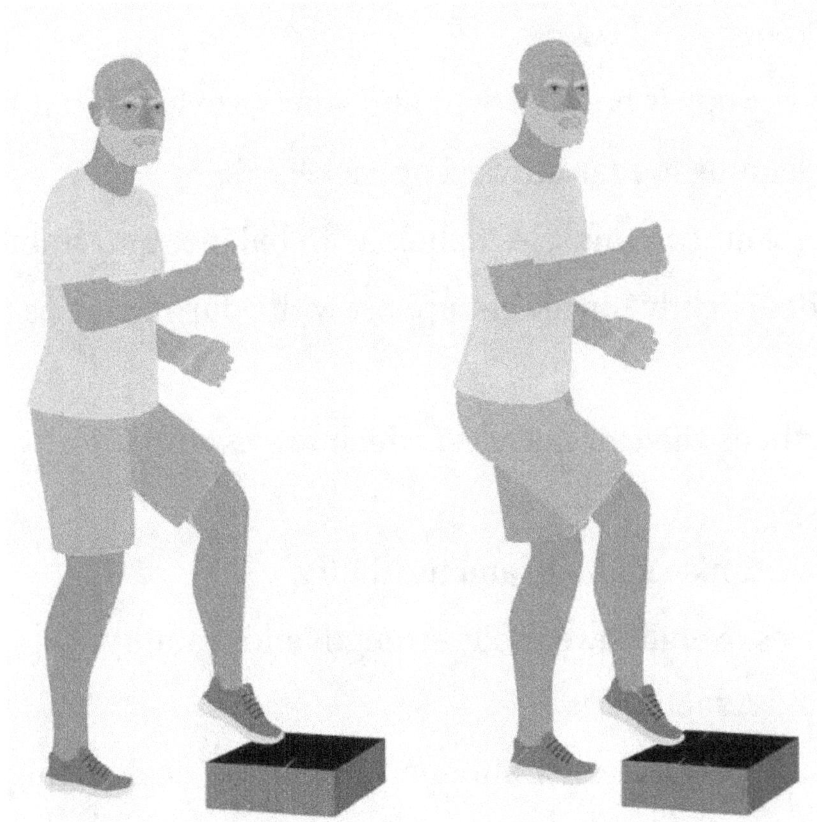

Exercise: Toe Taps

<u>Exercise: Heel Raises</u>

Objective of the Exercise: To strengthen the calf muscles and improve balance by performing heel raises.

Difficulty Level: Beginner

Equipment Needed: A sturdy chair or countertop for support

Detailed Description:

- Stand up straight, holding onto a sturdy chair or countertop for support.
- Place your feet shoulder-width apart.
- Raise your heels off the ground, lifting your body onto the balls of your feet.
- Hold the raised position for a moment, then slowly lower your heels back down to the ground.
- Repeat this movement for 10-12 repetitions.

Key Focus Points:

- Keep your upper body upright and your gaze forward throughout the exercise.
- Avoid leaning too far forward or backward.
- Engage your core muscles to help with balance and stability.
- If needed, lightly touch the support with your fingertips for stability.

Benefits:

- Strengthens the calf muscles, which are essential for walking and maintaining balance.
- Improves ankle stability and flexibility.
- Enhances overall lower body strength and stability.

Variations and Adaptations:

- If raising both heels simultaneously is too challenging, you can perform the exercise one leg at a time.
- You can also increase the difficulty by performing the heel raises on an unstable surface, such as a foam pad.

Frequency and Duration: Aim to perform this exercise for 10-12 repetitions, twice a day.

Exercise: Standing Hip Abduction

Objective of the Exercise: To strengthen the muscles in the hips and improve balance by performing standing hip abductions.

Difficulty Level: Beginner

Equipment Needed: A clear, open space

Detailed Description:

- Stand up straight with your feet hip-width apart and your arms by your sides.
- Shift your weight onto your right leg.
- Lift your left leg out to the side, keeping it straight and parallel to the ground.
- Hold the lifted position for a moment, then lower your left leg back down to the ground.

- Repeat this movement for 10-12 repetitions, then switch to the other leg.

Key Focus Points:

- Keep your upper body stable and your core engaged throughout the exercise.
- Avoid leaning to the side or tilting your body.
- Engage the muscles in the standing leg to help with balance and stability.
- If needed, lightly touch a support with your fingertips for stability.

Benefits:

- Strengthens the muscles in the hips, particularly the glutes and outer thighs.
- Improves balance and stability by challenging the muscles in the standing leg.
- Enhances overall lower body strength and stability.

Variations and Adaptations:

- If standing hip abductions are too challenging, you can perform the exercise while holding onto a support with one hand.
- You can also increase the difficulty by adding ankle weights or performing the abductions on an unstable surface, such as a foam pad.

Frequency and Duration: Aim to perform this exercise for 10-12 repetitions on each leg, twice a day.

Exercise: Marching in Place

Objective of the Exercise: To improve balance, coordination, and cardiovascular fitness by marching in place.

Difficulty Level: Beginner

Equipment Needed: A clear, open space

Detailed Description:

- Stand up straight with your feet hip-width apart and your arms by your sides.
- Lift your right knee up towards your chest, then lower it back down to the ground.
- Repeat this movement with your left knee, lifting it up towards your chest and lowering it back down.

- Continue alternating between the right and left knee, marching in place.

Key Focus Points:

- Keep your upper body upright and your gaze forward throughout the exercise.
- Engage your core muscles to help with balance and stability.
- Land softly on the balls of your feet with each march.
- Try to maintain a steady and controlled pace throughout the exercise.

Benefits:

- Improves balance, coordination, and cardiovascular fitness.
- Strengthens the muscles in the legs, particularly the quadriceps and hip flexors.
- Enhances overall lower body strength and stability.

Variations and Adaptations:

- If marching in place is too challenging, you can perform this exercise while holding onto a support with one hand.
- You can also increase the difficulty by adding ankle weights or marching at a faster pace.

Frequency and Duration: Aim to perform this exercise for 1-2 minutes, twice a day.

• INTERMEDIATE BALANCE CHALLENGES TO STIMULATE THE VESTIBULAR SYSTEM

Exercise 1: Tandem Walk

Objective of the Exercise: To improve balance and coordination by challenging the vestibular system during walking.

Difficulty Level: Intermediate

Equipment Needed: A clear and unobstructed space

Detailed Description:

- Find a straight pathway or hallway where you can walk without any obstacles.
- Stand with your feet together, arms relaxed at your sides.

- Take a step forward with your left foot, placing the heel directly in front of the toes of your right foot.
- Bring your right foot forward, placing it in front of the toes of your left foot.
- Continue walking in a straight line, placing one foot directly in front of the other.

Key Focus Points:

- Maintain a slow and steady pace, focusing on your balance and coordination.
- Keep your eyes focused straight ahead to engage the vestibular system effectively.
- Keep your core muscles engaged and your posture upright throughout the exercise.

Benefits:

- Improves balance and stability while walking, reducing the risk of tripping or falling.
- Challenges the vestibular system by requiring precise control of body movements.

Variations and Adaptations:

- If you find it challenging to maintain balance, use a wall or railing for support.
- For an increased challenge, try walking with your eyes closed, relying solely on your vestibular system for balance.

Frequency and Duration: Perform the tandem walk for 10-15 steps, twice a day.

Exercise 2: Standing Heel-to-Toe

Objective of the Exercise: To improve balance and proprioception by challenging the vestibular system and lower body stability.

Difficulty Level: Intermediate

Equipment Needed: A clear and unobstructed space

Detailed Description:

- Stand with your feet together, arms relaxed at your sides.

- Place the heel of your right foot directly in front of the toes of your left foot, touching them together.
- Focus on a fixed point in front of you to maintain balance.
- Slowly lift your right foot off the ground, balancing on your left foot with the heel and toes touching.
- Hold this position for a few seconds, then lower your right foot back down.
- Repeat the exercise, this time lifting your left foot off the ground.

Key Focus Points:

- Maintain a steady gaze on the fixed point to engage the vestibular system effectively.
- Keep your core muscles engaged and your posture upright throughout the exercise.
- If needed, lightly touch a wall or stable surface for support.

Benefits:

- Enhances balance and stability, particularly in challenging positions.
- Improves proprioception, the body's awareness of its position in space.

Variations and Adaptations:

- If you find it challenging to maintain balance, use a wall or railing for support.
- For an increased challenge, try closing your eyes while balancing on one foot.

Frequency and Duration: Perform 10 repetitions on each side, twice a day.

<u>Exercise 3: Clock Reach</u>

Objective of the Exercise: To improve balance and coordination by challenging the vestibular system through controlled movements.

Difficulty Level: Intermediate

Equipment Needed: A clear and unobstructed space

Detailed Description:

- Stand with your feet shoulder-width apart, arms relaxed at your sides.

- Imagine yourself standing in the center of a clock, with 12 o'clock directly in front of you and 6 o'clock behind you.
- Start by reaching your right arm directly in front of you towards 12 o'clock.
- Return your arm to the starting position, then reach towards 6 o'clock behind you.
- Repeat the exercise, this time reaching with your left arm towards 12 o'clock and then towards 6 o'clock.

Key Focus Points:

- Maintain proper posture throughout the exercise, keeping your shoulders relaxed and your chin parallel to the ground.
- Perform the reaches slowly and smoothly, focusing on your balance and coordination.
- Keep your eyes focused straight ahead to engage the vestibular system effectively.

Benefits:

- Challenges the vestibular system through controlled movements in different directions.
- Improves balance and coordination, reducing the risk of falls.

Variations and Adaptations:

- If you find it challenging to maintain balance, perform the exercise while seated on a stable chair.
- For an increased challenge, try closing your eyes while reaching in different directions.

Frequency and Duration: Perform 10 repetitions on each side, twice a day.

Exercise 4: Standing Knee Lifts

Objective of the Exercise: To improve balance and strengthen the hip flexor muscles, which play a crucial role in stability.

Difficulty Level: Intermediate

Equipment Needed: A sturdy chair without wheels

Detailed Description:

- Start by standing behind a sturdy chair, holding onto the back for support.
- Stand with your feet shoulder-width apart, arms relaxed at your sides.
- Shift your weight to your right leg, keeping your left foot slightly off the ground and with the toe pointing downwards.
- Slowly lift your left knee towards your chest, keeping your thigh parallel to the ground.
- Pause for a moment, then lower your left foot back down.
- Repeat the exercise, this time lifting your right knee towards your chest.

Key Focus Points:

- Maintain proper posture throughout the exercise, keeping your shoulders relaxed and your chin parallel to the ground.
- Perform the knee lifts slowly and smoothly, focusing on your balance and control.
- Keep your eyes focused straight ahead to engage the vestibular system effectively.

Benefits:

- Strengthens the hip flexor muscles, which are essential for balance and stability.
- Improves balance and coordination, reducing the risk of falls.

Variations and Adaptations:

- If you find it challenging to maintain balance, perform the knee lifts while seated on a stable chair.
- For an increased challenge, try closing your eyes while lifting your knee towards your chest.

Frequency and Duration: Perform 10 repetitions on each leg, twice a day.

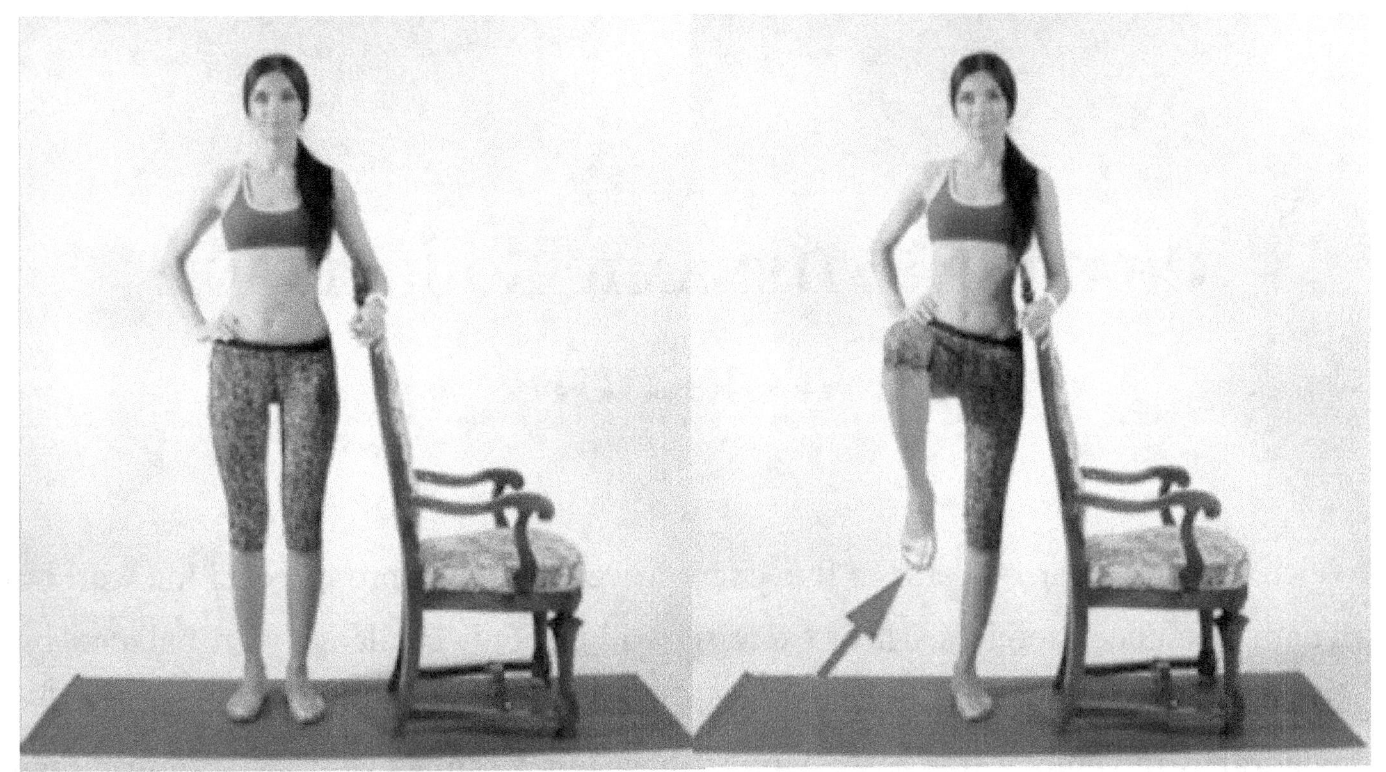

Exercise 4: Standing Knee Lifts

CHAPTER 8: DYNAMIC EQUILIBRIUM WORKOUTS

Welcome back, dear readers! In this chapter we will delve into the exciting world of dynamic balance exercises. These exercises will not only challenge your balance, but also improve your overall strength, coordination and flexibility. Get ready to feel invigorated and empowered as we explore these invigorating exercises! (Some of them you already know and will be able to perform with more experience than your first time)

EMBRACE THE POWER OF MOVEMENT

Life is all about movement, and our bodies are designed to be in motion. By engaging in dynamic equilibrium workouts, we can tap into the inherent power of movement and unlock our full potential. These exercises will not only keep you physically active but also stimulate your mind and boost your overall well-being.

As we age, our bodies naturally lose muscle mass and flexibility, which can affect our balance and increase the risk of falls. But fear not, my friends! Dynamic equilibrium workouts are here to save the day. By challenging our bodies in new and exciting ways, we can improve our balance, posture, and confidence.

STEP INTO ACTION

Let's kick things off with an exercise that will get your heart pumping and your muscles working. Stand tall with your feet hip-width apart, and imagine a tightrope stretched out in front of you. Now, take a step forward with your right foot, placing it directly in front of your left foot, as if you were walking on a tightrope.

As you step forward, engage your core muscles and maintain a steady pace. Feel the muscles in your legs and hips working together to keep you stable. Take a few more steps, alternating between your right and left foot. Remember to keep your gaze forward and your posture upright.

Next, let's move on to a side-to-side exercise that will challenge your balance and coordination. Stand with your feet shoulder-width apart, and imagine a line running from side to side. Shift your weight onto your right foot and lift your left foot slightly off the ground.

Now, step your left foot to the side, crossing over the imaginary line. As you do this, maintain your balance and keep your core engaged. Return to the starting position and repeat the movement on the other side. Feel the muscles in your legs and hips working together to keep you steady.

BALANCE AND BREATHE

Now that we've warmed up with some dynamic movements, let's focus on balance and breathing. Find a comfortable spot where you can stand with plenty of room around you. Stand tall with your feet hip-width apart and your arms relaxed at your sides.

Take a deep breath in through your nose, filling your lungs with air. As you exhale through your mouth, slowly lift one foot off the ground, bringing your knee up towards your chest. Hold this position for a few seconds, focusing on your balance and the sensation of your foot lifting off the ground.

Lower your foot back down to the ground and repeat the movement with the other leg. Remember to keep your gaze forward and your core engaged. Feel the muscles in your standing leg working to keep you stable.

CHALLENGE YOURSELF

As you become more comfortable with these dynamic equilibrium workouts, don't be afraid to challenge yourself. Try adding some variations to the exercises we've covered so far. For example, you can try walking on the tightrope while holding a lightweight object in each hand to increase the difficulty.

Remember, my dear readers, the key to success is consistency. Aim to incorporate these dynamic equilibrium workouts into your daily routine for just five minutes a day. Over time, you will notice improvements in your balance, posture, and overall confidence.

Well, my friends, that wraps up our exploration of dynamic equilibrium workouts. I hope you feel inspired and empowered to incorporate these exercises into your daily routine. Remember, maintaining your balance is not only about physical health but also about enhancing your overall well-being. Keep moving, stay motivated, and embrace the power of dynamic equilibrium!

• DYNAMIC EXERCISES TO CHALLENGE BALANCE AND COORDINATION

Exercise: Single Leg Stance

Objective of the Exercise: To improve balance and stability on one leg.

Difficulty Level: Beginner

Equipment Needed: A sturdy chair without wheels.

Detailed Description:

- Stand behind a chair, holding onto the back for support.
- Lift one foot off the ground, bending the knee slightly.
- Try to maintain your balance on the standing leg for as long as possible.
- If needed, lightly touch your toe to the ground for stability.

Key Focus Points:

- Keep your back straight and your core engaged.
- Focus your gaze on a fixed point in front of you to help with balance.
- Try to distribute your weight evenly on the standing leg.
- Don't forget to breathe throughout the exercise.

Benefits:

- Strengthens the muscles in the legs and ankles, improving stability.

- Enhances proprioception, which is the body's awareness of its position in space.
- Helps to prevent falls by improving balance and coordination.

Variations and Adaptations:

- If standing without support is too challenging, hold onto the chair with both hands.
- You can also perform this exercise with your eyes closed to further challenge your balance.

Frequency and Duration: Start with 10 seconds on each leg and gradually increase the duration as your balance improves. Aim for 3 sets on each leg, twice a day.

Exercise: Tandem Stand

Objective of the Exercise: To improve balance and stability while standing in a narrow base of support.

Difficulty Level: Intermediate

Equipment Needed: A clear, flat surface.

Detailed Description:

- Stand with your feet together, arms relaxed at your sides.
- Place one foot directly in front of the other, so that the heel of the front foot is touching the toes of the back foot.
- Engage your core muscles and maintain your balance in this position.
- Hold the position for as long as you can, then switch the position of your feet.

Key Focus Points:

- Keep your gaze focused straight ahead to maintain balance.
- Engage your core muscles to help stabilize your body.
- Try to distribute your weight evenly on both feet.
- Don't forget to breathe throughout the exercise.

Benefits:

- Improves balance and stability, particularly in a narrow base of support.

- Strengthens the muscles in the legs, ankles, and core.
- Enhances proprioception and body awareness.

Variations and Adaptations:

- If you have difficulty maintaining balance, you can perform this exercise while holding onto a wall or railing for support.
- For an added challenge, try closing your eyes while holding the tandem stand position.

Frequency and Duration: Start with 10 seconds in each position and gradually increase the duration as your balance improves. Aim for 3 sets in each position, twice a day.

Exercise: Hip Abduction

Objective of the Exercise: To strengthen the muscles in the hips and outer thighs, improving balance and stability.

Difficulty Level: Intermediate

Equipment Needed: A clear, flat surface.

Detailed Description:

- Stand with your feet hip-width apart, arms relaxed at your sides.
- Shift your weight onto your left leg and lift your right leg out to the side, keeping it straight.
- Lower your right leg back down to the starting position with control.
- Repeat the lifts for the desired number of repetitions, then switch to the other leg.

Key Focus Points:

- Keep your core engaged and your back straight throughout the exercise.
- Avoid leaning to the side or twisting your upper body.
- Focus on controlling the movement and maintaining your balance.
- Use your arms for balance if needed.

Benefits:

- Strengthens the muscles in the hips and outer thighs, improving stability.

- Enhances balance and coordination.
- Increases hip mobility and flexibility.

Variations and Adaptations:

- If standing without support is too challenging, hold onto a chair or wall for balance.
- You can also perform this exercise seated on a chair, lifting one leg out to the side at a time.

Frequency and Duration: Aim for 10-15 lifts on each leg, twice a day.

- **INTEGRATION OF DYNAMIC MOVEMENTS INTO DAILY ROUTINE**

Chair Sit-to-Stand

- **Objective of the Exercise:** To improve lower body strength and balance by simulating the movement of standing up from a chair.
- **Difficulty Level:** Beginner
- **Equipment Needed:** A sturdy chair without wheels
- **Detailed Description:**
  - Start by sitting in the middle of the chair, feet flat on the floor, and hip-width apart.
  - Place your hands on the armrests or on your thighs for support.
  - Lean slightly forward and push through your heels to stand up, keeping your back straight.
  - Once fully standing, pause for a moment, then slowly lower yourself back down to the chair in a controlled manner.
  - Repeat the movement for a set number of repetitions.
- **Key Focus Points:**
  - Engage your core and keep your back straight throughout the exercise.
  - Avoid using momentum; focus on using your leg muscles to stand up.

- Keep your weight evenly distributed between both legs.
  - Move slowly and control the descent to avoid plopping down into the chair.
- **Benefits:**
  - Strengthens the quadriceps, hamstrings, and glutes, which are essential for standing and walking.
  - Improves balance and coordination by simulating a daily activity.
  - Enhances overall lower body strength and endurance.
- **Variations and Adaptations:**
  - If standing up is difficult, start by using a chair with armrests to assist you.
  - For an added challenge, cross your arms over your chest during the exercise.
- **Frequency and Duration:** Aim to perform 10-15 sit-to-stands, twice a day.

Side Stepping

- **Objective of the Exercise:** To improve lateral stability and coordination by practicing controlled side-to-side movements.
- **Difficulty Level:** Intermediate
- **Equipment Needed:** A clear, open space
- **Detailed Description:**
  - Stand with your feet hip-width apart and arms relaxed by your sides.
  - Take a step to the right with your right foot, followed by your left foot, bringing your feet together.
  - Continue stepping to the right for a set number of steps, then switch direction and step to the left.
  - Focus on controlled movements and maintaining balance throughout the exercise.
- **Key Focus Points:**
  - Keep your body upright and avoid leaning to one side.
  - Engage your core and maintain a steady pace.

- Make sure your steps are controlled and deliberate, avoiding any jerky movements.
  - Use your arms for balance by gently swinging them in coordination with your steps.
- **Benefits:**
  - Strengthens the muscles on the sides of your hips and thighs.
  - Improves lateral stability, reducing the risk of falls during sideways movements.
  - Enhances overall coordination and balance.
- **Variations and Adaptations:**
  - If side stepping is difficult, start with smaller steps and gradually increase the width as you gain confidence.
  - Perform the exercise while holding onto a countertop or wall for added support if needed.
- **Frequency and Duration:** Aim to perform 10-15 side steps in each direction, twice a day.

Backward Walking

- **Objective of the Exercise:** To challenge balance and coordination by walking backward, a movement that is less commonly practiced.
- **Difficulty Level:** Intermediate
- **Equipment Needed:** A clear, open space
- **Detailed Description:**
  - Stand with your feet hip-width apart and arms relaxed by your sides.
  - Begin walking backward by stepping with your right foot, followed by your left, moving in a straight line.
  - Keep your gaze forward and your movements slow and controlled to maintain balance.
  - Continue walking backward for a set distance or number of steps.

- **Key Focus Points:**
    - Engage your core and maintain an upright posture throughout the exercise.
    - Take small, controlled steps to avoid losing balance.
    - Focus on a point in front of you to help maintain stability while moving backward.
    - Use your arms for balance, swinging them gently as you step.
- **Benefits:**
    - Improves balance and coordination, particularly in less familiar movements.
    - Strengthens the muscles in the legs and core.
    - Enhances spatial awareness and proprioception.
- **Variations and Adaptations:**
    - If walking backward is challenging, start by practicing near a wall or sturdy surface for added support.
    - Perform the exercise on a soft surface, such as a carpet, to reduce the impact if balance is lost.
- **Frequency and Duration:** Aim to walk backward for 10-15 steps, twice a day.

Figure-8 Walking

- **Objective of the Exercise:** To improve dynamic balance and coordination by walking in a figure-8 pattern.
- **Difficulty Level:** Intermediate
- **Equipment Needed:** A clear, open space with enough room to walk in a figure-8 shape
- **Detailed Description:**
    - Stand with your feet hip-width apart and arms relaxed by your sides.
    - Begin walking in a figure-8 pattern, taking small, controlled steps.

- Focus on maintaining a steady pace and smooth turns as you navigate the figure-8.
    - Continue walking in the figure-8 for a set amount of time or number of loops.
- **Key Focus Points:**
    - Engage your core and keep your body upright as you walk.
    - Focus on smooth, controlled turns as you change direction.
    - Keep your weight centered and avoid leaning to one side.
    - Use your arms for balance by gently swinging them in coordination with your steps.
- **Benefits:**
    - Enhances dynamic balance and stability during complex movements.
    - Strengthens the muscles in the lower body, including the legs and core.
    - Improves coordination and proprioception, reducing the risk of falls.
- **Variations and Adaptations:**
    - If walking in a figure-8 is challenging, start by walking in a simple circular pattern and gradually increase the complexity.
    - Perform the exercise near a wall or sturdy surface for added support if needed.
- **Frequency and Duration:** Aim to walk in the figure-8 pattern for 1-2 minutes, twice a day.

Hip Circles

- **Objective of the Exercise:** To improve hip mobility and balance by practicing controlled circular movements.
- **Difficulty Level:** Beginner
- **Equipment Needed:** A sturdy chair or wall for support
- **Detailed Description:**

- Stand with your feet hip-width apart and lightly hold onto a chair or wall for support.
- Shift your weight onto your right foot and lift your left foot slightly off the ground.
- Slowly move your left leg in a circular motion, making small circles with your hip.
- Complete a set number of circles, then switch to the other leg.

- **Key Focus Points:**
  - Engage your core and maintain an upright posture throughout the exercise.
  - Keep your movements slow and controlled, focusing on the circular motion.
  - Avoid leaning to one side or using your arms excessively for balance.
  - Focus on the smooth rotation of your hip joint.

- **Benefits:**
  - Improves hip mobility and flexibility, which are essential for balance and movement.
  - Strengthens the muscles around the hip joint.
  - Enhances overall coordination and stability.

- **Variations and Adaptations:**
  - If balancing on one leg is difficult, start by performing the exercise with your foot lightly touching the ground.
  - Increase the size of the circles as you gain confidence and control.

- **Frequency and Duration:** Aim to perform 10-15 hip circles on each leg, twice a day.

As you continue on your journey to improve your balance, posture, and confidence, it is important to incorporate progression strategies into your dynamic equilibrium training. These strategies will help you challenge yourself and continue to make progress in your balance exercises.

1. INCREASE DURATION

One way to progress in your dynamic equilibrium training is to gradually increase the duration of your exercises. Start by performing each exercise for 30 seconds, and as you become more comfortable and confident, gradually increase the duration to one minute or longer. This will help improve your endurance and stability.

2. ADD VARIATIONS

To further challenge your balance, consider adding variations to your exercises. For example, you can perform the single-leg stand with your eyes closed or try standing on an unstable surface, such as a foam pad or a balance disc. These variations will engage different muscles and force your body to work harder to maintain balance.

3. INCREASE DIFFICULTY

Once you have mastered the basic exercises, it's time to increase the difficulty level. You can do this by adding resistance, such as holding light weights or using resistance bands, to your exercises. This will not only challenge your balance but also help improve your strength and stability.

4. INCORPORATE DYNAMIC MOVEMENTS

Balance exercises don't have to be static. Incorporating dynamic movements into your training can help improve your balance in real-life situations. For example, you can try walking heel-to-toe in a straight line, performing side steps, or even practicing Tai Chi.

These movements will challenge your balance in different ways and help improve your overall stability and coordination.

5. PROGRESS TO UNILATERAL EXERCISES

Once you feel comfortable with bilateral exercises, such as the single-leg stand, you can progress to unilateral exercises. These exercises involve balancing on one leg at a time and are more challenging for your balance. Examples of unilateral exercises include the single-leg deadlift, the single-leg squat, and the single-leg balance reach. Start with a stable surface and gradually progress to an unstable surface for an added challenge.

6. INCREASE FREQUENCY

Lastly, to continue making progress in your dynamic equilibrium training, consider increasing the frequency of your exercises. Aim to incorporate balance exercises into your daily routine, ideally for at least five minutes a day. Consistency is key when it comes to improving your balance, so make it a habit to prioritize your balance exercises.

Remember, always listen to your body and progress at a pace that feels comfortable for you. If you experience any pain or discomfort, it's important to consult with a healthcare professional. By incorporating these progression strategies into your dynamic equilibrium training, you will continue to improve your balance, posture, and confidence, ultimately enhancing your overall well-being and quality of life.

Chapter 9: Mind-Body Connection

As we age, it's essential to recognize the profound connection between our minds and bodies. Our mental state can directly impact our physical well-being, and vice versa. In this chapter, we will explore the powerful mind-body connection and how it relates to balance, posture, and overall health.

The Power of Positive Thinking

Our thoughts have a significant influence on our actions and physical abilities. When we approach balance exercises with a positive mindset, we are more likely to succeed. Negative thoughts and self-doubt can hinder our progress and make us more susceptible to falls. Therefore, it's crucial to cultivate a positive attitude towards our exercises.

Imagine yourself confidently performing each exercise, feeling strong and balanced. Visualize yourself achieving your goals and maintaining your independence. This positive mental imagery can help improve your overall performance and motivation.

Stress and Its Impact on Balance

Stress can have a detrimental effect on our balance and posture. When we are stressed, our muscles tense up, and our bodies become more rigid. This tension can throw off our balance and increase the risk of falls.

Engaging in relaxation techniques, such as deep breathing exercises or meditation, can help reduce stress levels and improve our balance. By incorporating these practices into our daily routine, we can enhance our mind-body connection and promote a sense of calmness and stability.

The Role of Mindfulness

Mindfulness is the practice of being fully present in the moment. By focusing our attention on the present, we can improve our balance and body awareness. When performing balance exercises, it's crucial to concentrate on the sensations in our bodies and the movements we are making.

Pay attention to how your weight shifts, how your muscles engage, and how your body responds to each movement. This mindful approach allows us to make subtle adjustments and maintain our balance more effectively.

Visualization Techniques

Visualization is a powerful tool that can enhance our performance and confidence. Before starting your balance exercises, take a moment to visualize yourself successfully completing each movement. See yourself standing tall, feeling stable, and maintaining your balance with ease.

By incorporating visualization into our exercise routine, we can train our minds to believe in our abilities, improving our overall performance and reducing the fear of falling.

The Importance of Relaxation

Relaxation is crucial for both our physical and mental well-being. When we are tense, our muscles become rigid, making it more challenging to maintain balance. Incorporating relaxation exercises, such as gentle stretching or progressive muscle relaxation, can help release tension and improve our overall balance.

Take time each day to engage in activities that promote relaxation and stress relief. This could be listening to calming music, practicing deep breathing exercises, or enjoying a warm bath. By prioritizing relaxation, we can enhance our mind-body connection and improve our overall balance and well-being.

The mind-body connection is a powerful tool in maintaining balance, posture, and overall health. By cultivating a positive mindset, managing stress, practicing mindfulness, and incorporating relaxation techniques, we can enhance our physical abilities and reduce the risk of falls.

Remember, our thoughts and mental state play a significant role in our physical well-being. Embrace the power of the mind-body connection and empower yourself to maintain an active, independent lifestyle.

• MINDFULNESS AND MEDITATION PRACTICES FOR IMPROVED BALANCE

Mindfulness and meditation practices are not only beneficial for mental well-being but also play a crucial role in improving balance and stability. By incorporating these practices into your daily routine, you can enhance your overall sense of body awareness, reduce stress, and promote a greater sense of calm and focus. In this chapter, we will explore various mindfulness and meditation techniques that can help you improve your balance and posture.

THE POWER OF MINDFULNESS

Mindfulness is the practice of being fully present in the moment, without judgment or attachment to thoughts, emotions, or sensations. It involves paying attention to your body, breath, and surroundings, cultivating a sense of awareness and acceptance. By practicing mindfulness, you can develop a deeper connection with your body, which is essential for improving balance.

Important: Mindfulness can help you become more aware of any imbalances or asymmetries in your body, allowing you to address and correct them.

BODY SCAN MEDITATION

One powerful mindfulness practice that can help improve balance is the body scan meditation. This practice involves systematically bringing your attention to different parts of your body, noticing any sensations, tension, or discomfort. By cultivating a non-judgmental awareness of your body, you can become more attuned to subtle changes in balance and posture.

Important: The body scan meditation can help you identify areas of tension or weakness that may be affecting your balance and stability.

BREATHING EXERCISES

Deep, diaphragmatic breathing is an essential component of mindfulness and can significantly impact your balance. When you take slow, deep breaths, you activate your diaphragm and engage your core muscles, promoting stability and improving posture. Important: Incorporating deep breathing exercises into your daily routine can help you maintain a strong and stable core, which is crucial for balance.

WALKING MEDITATION

Walking meditation is a mindfulness practice that involves bringing your attention to the sensations of walking. It can be done indoors or outdoors, at a slow and deliberate pace. By focusing on the movement of your feet, the shifting of your weight, and the sensations in your body, you can improve your balance and body awareness. Important: Walking meditation can help you develop a more grounded and stable connection with the earth, enhancing your overall balance and stability.

VISUALIZATION TECHNIQUES

Visualization is a powerful tool that can help improve balance by training your mind to create mental images of stability and strength. By visualizing yourself in a balanced and steady posture, you can reinforce positive neural pathways and improve your body's ability to maintain balance. Important: Visualization techniques can be particularly helpful for individuals who may have physical limitations that prevent them from performing certain balance exercises.

TAI CHI AND QIGONG

Tai Chi and Qigong are ancient Chinese practices that combine movement, breath control, and mindfulness. These practices promote balance, flexibility, and overall well-being. By incorporating Tai Chi or Qigong into your routine, you can improve your balance, posture, and body awareness.

Important: Tai Chi and Qigong are gentle exercises that can be modified to suit individuals of all fitness levels and abilities.

By incorporating mindfulness and meditation practices into your daily routine, you can enhance your balance, posture, and overall well-being. These practices not only improve your physical stability but also promote a sense of calm, focus, and body awareness. Take a few minutes each day to practice mindfulness and experience the transformative benefits it can have on your balance and confidence.

• VISUALIZATION TECHNIQUES FOR ENHANCING STABILITY AND CONFIDENCE

Visualization techniques can be powerful tools for enhancing stability and confidence, especially when it comes to balance exercises for seniors. By using the power of the mind to create mental images, seniors can improve their ability to perform exercises correctly and with greater ease. This chapter will explore various visualization techniques that can be incorporated into daily balance exercises.

1. CENTERING VISUALIZATION

Begin by finding a quiet and comfortable space to practice this visualization technique. Close your eyes and take a few deep breaths to relax your body and mind. Imagine a strong and stable center within your body, located just below your navel. Visualize this center as a glowing ball of light, radiating warmth and strength.

As you continue to visualize this center, imagine that it extends downward into the ground, connecting you to the earth's stability. Feel the support and grounding provided by this connection. Now, imagine that the light from your center expands outward, filling your entire body with a sense of stability and balance.

Hold this visualization for a few moments, allowing yourself to fully embody the feeling of being centered and stable. When you're ready, open your eyes and proceed with your balance exercises, carrying this sense of stability with you.

2. Tree Visualization

This visualization technique draws inspiration from the strength and stability of a tree. Stand tall with your feet hip-width apart, imagining that your feet are firmly rooted into the ground like the roots of a tree. Feel the stability and support provided by your rooted feet.

Visualize your body growing upward, just like the trunk of a tree. Imagine your spine lengthening and your posture improving as you reach towards the sky. Picture your arms and legs as branches, extending outwards with grace and strength.

As you practice your balance exercises, imagine that you are swaying gently in the breeze, just like the branches of a tree. Embrace the feeling of being grounded, stable, and connected to the earth.

3. Tightrope Visualization

This visualization technique can be particularly helpful for improving balance. Imagine yourself walking along a tightrope, high above the ground. Visualize the tightrope as a thin line stretching out in front of you, with your arms extended to the sides for balance.

As you walk along the tightrope, focus on maintaining a steady and controlled movement. Imagine that you are engaging your core muscles to stay balanced, just like a tightrope walker. Keep your gaze fixed straight ahead, focusing on a point in the distance.

As you continue to practice your balance exercises, incorporate this visualization to enhance your stability and confidence. Embrace the feeling of being poised and in control, just like a skilled tightrope walker.

4. Beach Visualization

This visualization technique taps into the calming and soothing qualities of the beach. Find a quiet space where you can sit comfortably. Close your eyes and take a few deep breaths to relax.

Visualize yourself sitting on a beautiful beach, with the sound of gentle waves in the background. Feel the warmth of the sun on your skin and the softness of the sand beneath you. Picture yourself standing up and walking along the shore, with each step feeling steady and balanced.

As you practice your balance exercises, imagine that you are still on the beach, surrounded by the serene environment. Allow the peacefulness of the beach to flow through your body, enhancing your stability and confidence.

5. MIRROR VISUALIZATION

This visualization technique focuses on improving posture and alignment. Stand in front of a mirror, with your feet hip-width apart. Take a moment to observe your current posture, noting any areas of imbalance or misalignment.

Begin to visualize your body aligning itself with the mirror image, creating a symmetrical and balanced posture. Imagine that your spine is lengthening, your shoulders are relaxed, and your head is held high. Picture yourself standing tall and confident.

As you practice your balance exercises, continue to use the mirror visualization to guide your posture and alignment. Embrace the feeling of being poised and aligned, knowing that you are improving your balance and overall well-being.

By incorporating these visualization techniques into your balance exercises, you can enhance your stability and confidence. Remember to practice them regularly and allow yourself to fully engage with the mental images created. With consistent practice, you will not only improve your balance but also cultivate a sense of empowerment and well-being.

• RELAXATION AND STRESS REDUCTION METHODS

In this chapter, we will explore various relaxation and stress reduction methods that can help seniors improve their overall well-being. As we age, it becomes increasingly important to find ways to manage stress and promote relaxation, as these factors can greatly impact our physical and mental health. By incorporating these simple techniques into your daily routine, you can experience a greater sense of calm and peace.

BREATHING EXERCISES

Deep breathing exercises are a powerful tool for relaxation and stress reduction. By focusing on your breath, you can activate the body's natural relaxation response and calm your mind. To practice deep breathing, find a quiet and comfortable space. Sit or lie down in a relaxed position, close your eyes, and take a deep breath in through your nose. Feel your abdomen expand as you inhale, and then slowly exhale through your mouth, allowing any tension to leave your body. Repeat this process several times, focusing on the sensation of your breath.

MEDITATION

Meditation is a practice that involves focusing your attention and eliminating the stream of thoughts that may be causing stress or anxiety. It is a powerful tool for promoting relaxation and improving overall well-being. To start a meditation practice, find a quiet and peaceful space where you can sit comfortably. Close your eyes and bring your attention to your breath or a specific point of focus, such as a word or phrase. Allow any thoughts or distractions to pass by without judgment, gently bringing your attention back to your breath or point of focus. Start with just a few minutes each day and gradually increase the duration as you become more comfortable with the practice.

PROGRESSIVE MUSCLE RELAXATION

Progressive muscle relaxation is a technique that involves tensing and then relaxing different muscle groups in your body. By systematically tensing and releasing muscle groups, you can release physical tension and promote a sense of relaxation. To practice progressive muscle relaxation, find a comfortable position and close your eyes. Start with your toes and gradually work your way up your body, tensing and then relaxing each muscle group. Pay attention to the sensations in your body as you release tension, allowing yourself to fully relax.

GUIDED IMAGERY

Guided imagery is a relaxation technique that involves using your imagination to create a calming and peaceful mental image. By visualizing a serene and tranquil scene, you can promote relaxation and reduce stress. To practice guided imagery, find a quiet space where you can sit or lie down comfortably. Close your eyes and imagine yourself in a peaceful setting, such as a beach or a garden. Engage your senses by imagining the sights, sounds, and smells of this place. Allow yourself to fully immerse in this mental image, focusing on the sensations of relaxation and calm.

JOURNALING

Journaling is a therapeutic practice that can help seniors process their thoughts and emotions, reducing stress and promoting self-reflection. By writing down your thoughts and feelings, you can gain clarity and perspective on challenging situations. To start a journaling practice, find a quiet and comfortable space. Set aside a few minutes each day to write freely, without judgment or expectation. Explore your thoughts and emotions, and allow yourself to express them on paper. You may choose to write about specific experiences, or simply let your thoughts flow.

Incorporating relaxation and stress reduction methods into your daily routine can have a profound impact on your overall well-being. By practicing deep breathing, meditation, progressive muscle relaxation, guided imagery, and journaling, you can reduce stress, promote relaxation, and enhance your quality of life. Remember to take time for yourself each day and prioritize self-care. By nurturing your mind and body, you can maintain a sense of balance and find peace in your daily life.

Chapter 10: Motivational Approach and Positive Mindset

As we continue our journey towards improving balance, posture, and confidence, it's essential to address the mental aspect of our well-being. Our mindset plays a crucial role in our ability to stay motivated and committed to our exercise routine. In this chapter, we will explore the power of a motivational approach and how cultivating a positive mindset can enhance our progress.

The Power of Motivation

Staying motivated can be challenging, especially when faced with the inevitable ups and downs of life. However, by understanding the importance of motivation and adopting strategies to maintain it, we can overcome obstacles and continue on our path towards better balance and overall well-being.

Important: Motivation is the driving force that propels us forward, even when faced with difficulties. It is what keeps us committed to our exercise routine, allowing us to reap the benefits of improved balance, posture, and confidence.

Setting Meaningful Goals

One way to stay motivated is by setting meaningful goals. When we have a clear vision of what we want to achieve, it becomes easier to stay focused and committed. However, it's important to set realistic and attainable goals that align with our capabilities and current physical condition.

Important: Setting goals provides us with a sense of purpose and direction. It gives us something to strive for and helps us measure our progress along the way.

CELEBRATING SMALL VICTORIES

While it's essential to have long-term goals, it's equally important to celebrate the small victories along the way. Each time we complete an exercise or notice an improvement in our balance or posture, we should acknowledge and celebrate our achievements.

Important: Celebrating small victories boosts our confidence and reinforces our motivation. It reminds us of the progress we have made and encourages us to keep pushing forward.

POSITIVE SELF-TALK

Our internal dialogue has a significant impact on our mindset and motivation. By practicing positive self-talk, we can cultivate a more supportive and encouraging mindset. Instead of focusing on our limitations or setbacks, we should remind ourselves of our strengths and the progress we have made.

Important: Positive self-talk helps us overcome self-doubt and negative thinking. It allows us to approach our exercises with confidence and optimism, increasing our chances of success.

SEEKING SUPPORT

Having a support system can make a world of difference in our journey towards better balance and overall well-being. Whether it's a friend, family member, or a community of like-minded individuals, having someone to share our challenges and successes with can provide the motivation and encouragement we need to stay on track.

Important: Seeking support creates accountability and fosters a sense of belonging. It reminds us that we are not alone in our journey and that there are others who understand and support our goals.

By adopting a motivational approach and cultivating a positive mindset, we can enhance our progress in improving balance, posture, and confidence. Remember, motivation is not a constant state but a skill that can be developed and nurtured. With the right mindset and support, we can overcome any challenges that come our way and continue on our path towards a healthier and more fulfilling life.

Having a positive outlook is essential for long-term success in any endeavor, and improving balance and posture is no exception. The mind-body connection plays a significant role in our overall well-being, and cultivating a positive mindset can greatly enhance our ability to achieve our goals. In this chapter, we will explore some strategies to help you cultivate a positive outlook as you work towards improving your balance, posture, and overall health.

1. Practice Gratitude

Gratitude is a powerful tool that can shift our focus from what is lacking in our lives to what we already have. Take a few moments each day to reflect on the things you are grateful for. It could be as simple as appreciating the beauty of nature, the support of loved ones, or the ability to engage in daily activities. By acknowledging and expressing gratitude, you can reframe your mindset and foster a more positive outlook.

2. Set Realistic Goals

Setting realistic goals is crucial for maintaining motivation and a positive mindset. Start by identifying specific, achievable goals related to improving your balance and posture. Break down these goals into smaller, manageable steps that you can work on each day. Celebrate your progress along the way, no matter how small, and use it as fuel to keep moving forward. Remember, every step counts!

3. Surround Yourself with Supportive People

Having a strong support system can make a world of difference in your journey towards better balance and posture. Surround yourself with friends, family, or fellow seniors who share your goals and can provide encouragement and motivation. Joining a local exercise group or participating in online communities can also connect you with like-minded individuals who can offer support and share their experiences.

4. Practice Mindfulness

Mindfulness is the practice of being fully present in the moment, without judgment. By cultivating mindfulness, you can develop a greater awareness of your body, thoughts, and emotions. Incorporate mindfulness exercises into your daily routine, such as deep breathing, body scans, or guided meditations. These practices can help you stay grounded, reduce stress, and maintain a positive outlook as you engage in your balance and posture exercises.

5. Celebrate Small Victories

As you progress in your balance and posture exercises, it's important to celebrate even the smallest victories. Whether it's holding a balance pose for a few seconds longer or noticing improvements in your posture, take the time to acknowledge and celebrate these achievements. Rewarding yourself for your efforts will reinforce positive behavior and motivate you to continue striving for long-term success.

6. Stay Persistent and Patient

Improving balance and posture takes time and consistent effort. It's important to stay persistent and patient with yourself throughout the process. Understand that progress may not always be linear, and there may be setbacks along the way. Instead of getting discouraged, view these setbacks as opportunities for growth and learning. Stay committed to your daily exercises and maintain a positive outlook, knowing that every step you take is bringing you closer to your goals.

By incorporating these strategies into your daily routine, you can cultivate a positive outlook that will support your long-term success in improving your balance, posture, and overall well-being. Remember, your mindset is a powerful tool, and with a positive attitude, you can achieve remarkable results.

Setting realistic goals and celebrating progress are essential steps in any journey towards improving balance, posture, and overall well-being. By establishing achievable objectives and acknowledging achievements along the way, seniors can stay motivated and maintain a positive mindset throughout their exercise routine.

1. UNDERSTANDING THE IMPORTANCE OF REALISTIC GOALS

When it comes to balance exercises, setting realistic goals is crucial. It's important to remember that progress may be gradual, and it's essential to avoid setting unrealistic expectations that could lead to frustration or discouragement. By setting achievable goals, seniors can experience a sense of accomplishment and stay motivated to continue their exercise routine.

Here are some key points to consider when setting realistic goals:

- Start with small, manageable goals: Begin with exercises that are within your current abilities and gradually increase the difficulty level over time.
- Be specific: Clearly define what you want to achieve, whether it's improving balance, posture, or overall confidence.
- Consider your current limitations: Take into account any existing health conditions or physical limitations when setting goals.
- Consult with a healthcare professional: If you have any concerns or questions about setting realistic goals, it's always a good idea to seek guidance from a healthcare professional.

2. CELEBRATING PROGRESS AND STAYING MOTIVATED

Celebrating progress is an essential part of the journey towards improving balance and overall well-being. By acknowledging achievements, seniors can stay motivated and maintain a positive mindset throughout their exercise routine.

Here are some strategies for celebrating progress and staying motivated:

- Keep a progress journal: Document your achievements, no matter how small they may seem. This will serve as a reminder of your progress and provide motivation to keep going.
- Reward yourself: Treat yourself to small rewards for reaching milestones or accomplishing goals. It could be something as simple as enjoying a favorite activity or indulging in a special treat.
- Share your progress with others: Whether it's with a friend, family member, or a support group, sharing your achievements can help boost motivation and provide a sense of accountability.
- Visualize your goals: Create a mental image of what you want to achieve and visualize yourself successfully completing your balance exercises. This can help reinforce your motivation and focus.

Remember, every step forward is a step towards improved balance, posture, and overall well-being. By setting realistic goals and celebrating progress, seniors can stay motivated and continue on their path to a healthier, more confident lifestyle.

• INCORPORATING ENJOYABLE ACTIVITIES INTO EXERCISE ROUTINE

As we age, it becomes increasingly important to prioritize our physical health and well-being. Regular exercise is a key component of maintaining a healthy lifestyle, but it can often feel like a chore or something we have to force ourselves to do. However, exercise doesn't have to be boring or monotonous. In fact, incorporating enjoyable activities into our exercise routine can make it more engaging and sustainable in the long run.

1. Find activities you love: One of the best ways to make exercise more enjoyable is to choose activities that you genuinely love. Think about the things you enjoy doing, whether it's dancing, gardening, swimming, or playing a sport. By incorporating these activities into your exercise routine, you'll be more motivated to stick with it and have fun while doing it.

2. Exercise with a friend: Exercising with a friend or a group can make the experience more enjoyable and social. Not only will you have someone to chat with and share your progress, but it can also provide a sense of accountability and support. Consider joining a local senior fitness class or inviting a friend to go on regular walks or bike rides together.

3. Listen to music or audiobooks: Music has a powerful impact on our mood and can make exercise more enjoyable. Create a playlist of your favorite songs or listen to audiobooks or podcasts while exercising. Not only will it make the time go by faster, but it can also distract you from any discomfort or fatigue you may feel.

4. Explore outdoor activities: Taking your exercise routine outdoors can provide a change of scenery and make it more enjoyable. Consider going for a hike, taking a bike ride, or practicing yoga in a park. Not only will you get the benefits of physical activity, but you'll also be able to enjoy the beauty of nature and fresh air.

5. Make it a social activity: Exercise doesn't have to be a solitary activity. Consider joining a walking or hiking group, participating in a dance class, or playing a team sport. Not only will you get the physical benefits of exercise, but you'll also have the opportunity to socialize and make new friends.

6. Set goals and track your progress: Setting goals and tracking your progress can make exercise more enjoyable and rewarding. Start by setting realistic and achievable goals, such as increasing your daily step count or improving your flexibility. Use a fitness tracker or a simple journal to track your progress and celebrate your achievements along the way.

7. Mix it up: Doing the same exercise routine day after day can quickly become boring. To keep things interesting, try mixing up your activities. Incorporate a variety of exercises, such as strength training, balance exercises, cardiovascular activities, and

flexibility exercises. This not only keeps your body challenged but also keeps your mind engaged.

8. Reward yourself: Don't forget to reward yourself for sticking to your exercise routine. Treat yourself to a relaxing massage, a new workout outfit, or a favorite healthy snack. By rewarding yourself, you'll create positive associations with exercise and be more motivated to continue.

Remember, the key to incorporating enjoyable activities into your exercise routine is to find what works for you. Experiment with different activities and approaches until you find something that you genuinely enjoy and look forward to. By making exercise fun and enjoyable, you'll be more likely to stick with it and reap the many benefits it offers.

Take a break because I would like to give you **two 'Premium Content Bonuses'** that I promised you at the beginning of the book cover. They are: **Weekly Workout Routine Plan** and **Detailed Progress Tracker**.

To receive them simply scan the QR code below

(**or** log on to the internet and type into your browser this link
https://bit.ly/Balanceexercisesforseniors_BONUS)

Once you've downloaded your 2 free bonuses, you'll be able to feel more confident, more fitter and younger thanks to a **personalised Weekly Workout Routine Plan** and **Detailed Progress Tracker.**

What are you waiting for, download the 2 free BONUSES now!

Chapter 11: Customizing Your Workout Plan

Now that you have learned a variety of balance exercises in the previous chapters, it's time to create a workout plan that suits your individual needs and preferences. Customizing your workout plan will not only make it more enjoyable but also increase your motivation to stick with it. Remember, consistency is key when it comes to improving your balance, posture, and overall well-being.

Assess Your Current Fitness Level

Before customizing your workout plan, it's important to assess your current fitness level. This will help you determine where to start and how to progress gradually. Take a moment to evaluate your balance, strength, and flexibility. Be honest with yourself and don't push beyond your limits.

Important: If you have any existing health issues or concerns, it's always a good idea to consult with your healthcare provider before starting a new exercise program.

Set Realistic Goals

Setting realistic goals is crucial for staying motivated and tracking your progress. Think about what you want to achieve with your balance exercises. Do you want to improve your balance to feel more confident during daily activities? Or do you have specific goals, such as preventing falls or combating osteoporosis?

Important: Remember that progress takes time, and it's important to be patient with yourself. Start with small, achievable goals and gradually increase the intensity and duration of your exercises as you feel comfortable.

CHOOSE EXERCISES THAT SUIT YOU

With a wide range of balance exercises to choose from, it's essential to select the ones that suit your needs and preferences. Consider your fitness level, any physical limitations, and what exercises you enjoy the most. Remember, the best exercise routine is the one that you will stick to consistently.

Important: If you're unsure which exercises are suitable for you, refer back to the previous chapters for detailed instructions and modifications. Don't hesitate to reach out to a qualified fitness professional for guidance and support.

CREATE A SCHEDULE

Now that you have chosen your exercises, it's time to create a schedule that works for you. Aim for at least five minutes of balance exercises every day, but feel free to increase the duration as you progress. Consistency is key, so find a time of day that works best for you and make it a non-negotiable part of your routine.

Important: Consider incorporating your balance exercises into your existing daily activities. For example, you can do some exercises while brushing your teeth or waiting for the kettle to boil. This will help you integrate your workout seamlessly into your day.

TRACK YOUR PROGRESS

Tracking your progress is essential for staying motivated and celebrating your achievements. Keep a journal or use a fitness app to record your workouts, noting the exercises you did, the duration, and any observations or improvements you notice. This will not only help you stay accountable but also provide a sense of accomplishment as you see your progress over time.

Important: Don't forget to reassess your fitness level periodically to gauge your improvement and adjust your workout plan accordingly. Celebrate every milestone, no matter how small!

Customizing your workout plan is an exciting step towards improving your balance, posture, and confidence. By assessing your fitness level, setting realistic goals, choosing exercises that suit you, creating a schedule, and tracking your progress, you are setting yourself up for success. Remember, this journey is about taking small steps every day to enhance your overall well-being and maintain your independence. You've got this!

• TAILORING EXERCISES TO INDIVIDUAL NEEDS AND ABILITIES

When it comes to balance exercises for seniors, it's important to remember that one size does not fit all. Each person has unique needs and abilities, and it's crucial to tailor the exercises to match them. By doing so, you can ensure that the exercises are safe, effective, and enjoyable for each individual. Here are some key considerations for tailoring balance exercises:

1. ASSESSING INDIVIDUAL BALANCE AND STRENGTH

Before starting any exercise program, it's essential to assess an individual's balance and strength. This can be done through simple tests or by consulting with a healthcare professional. By understanding their current abilities, you can determine which exercises will be most beneficial and appropriate for them.

2. MODIFYING EXERCISES FOR DIFFERENT FITNESS LEVELS

Not everyone will have the same level of fitness or mobility. Some individuals may be beginners, while others may have been exercising regularly for years. It's important to provide modifications for each exercise to accommodate different fitness levels. For example, you can offer variations that make an exercise easier or more challenging, depending on the individual's needs.

3. Considering Existing Health Conditions

Seniors may have various health conditions that need to be taken into account when designing their exercise program. For instance, individuals with osteoporosis may need to avoid high-impact exercises that could increase the risk of fractures. By understanding and considering any existing health conditions, you can modify exercises or recommend alternative ones that are safe and suitable.

4. Incorporating Personal Interests

One way to make balance exercises more engaging and enjoyable is by incorporating personal interests. For example, if an individual enjoys dancing, you can include dance-inspired movements as part of their exercise routine. By aligning the exercises with their interests, it can help increase motivation and adherence to the program.

5. Providing Clear Instructions and Demonstrations

When explaining the exercises, it's important to provide clear instructions and demonstrations. Since the book does not include visual aids, it's crucial to use vivid and descriptive language to help readers visualize the movements. Step-by-step instructions should be provided for each exercise, ensuring that readers can safely perform them without needing illustrations.

6. Encouraging Regular Progression

As individuals become more comfortable with the exercises, it's important to encourage regular progression. This can involve gradually increasing the difficulty or intensity of the exercises over time. By doing so, seniors can continue to challenge themselves and make progress in improving their balance and overall well-being.

7. Offering Support and Adaptations

Lastly, it's essential to offer ongoing support and adaptations as needed. Some individuals may encounter difficulties or have questions along the way. By being available to address their concerns and provide adaptations, you can ensure that they feel supported throughout their exercise journey.

Remember, tailoring balance exercises to individual needs and abilities is key to creating a safe, effective, and enjoyable exercise program for seniors. By considering their unique circumstances and providing appropriate modifications, you can help them improve their balance, posture, and confidence, ultimately enhancing their overall quality of life.

• ADAPTING WORKOUTS FOR SPECIFIC HEALTH CONDITIONS

As we age, it's common to develop health conditions that may impact our ability to exercise. However, it's important to remember that physical activity can still be beneficial, even with certain health conditions. In this chapter, we will explore how to adapt workouts for specific health conditions, ensuring that everyone can safely and effectively improve their balance and posture.

OSTEOPOROSIS

Osteoporosis is a condition characterized by weak and brittle bones, making individuals more susceptible to fractures. If you have osteoporosis, it's crucial to choose exercises that are safe for your condition. Avoid high-impact activities that may increase the risk of fractures, such as jumping or running. Instead, focus on exercises that improve balance and strengthen muscles without putting excessive stress on the bones.

Recommended exercises for individuals with osteoporosis include:

- Heel-to-Toe Walk: This exercise helps improve balance and coordination. Stand with your feet in a straight line, placing one foot directly in front of the other. Take small steps, placing your heel in front of your toes with each step. Repeat for 10 steps, then switch feet.
- Wall Push-Ups: This exercise strengthens the upper body without putting stress on the wrists or spine. Stand facing a wall, about an arm's length away. Place your hands on the wall at shoulder height, slightly wider than shoulder-width apart. Slowly bend your elbows, lowering your chest towards the wall. Push back up to the starting position. Repeat for 10 repetitions.

- Chair Squats: This exercise strengthens the lower body and improves balance. Stand in front of a sturdy chair with your feet hip-width apart. Slowly lower your hips towards the chair, as if you were about to sit down. Just before touching the chair, engage your leg muscles and push back up to a standing position. Repeat for 10 repetitions.

ARTHRITIS

Arthritis is a common condition that causes joint pain and stiffness. If you have arthritis, it's important to choose exercises that are gentle on the joints and avoid activities that cause pain. Focus on low-impact exercises that improve flexibility, strengthen muscles, and reduce joint stiffness.

Recommended exercises for individuals with arthritis include:

- Neck Rotations: This exercise helps improve neck mobility and relieve tension. Sit or stand with your back straight. Slowly turn your head to the right, trying to bring your chin over your shoulder. Hold for a few seconds, then return to the center. Repeat on the left side. Perform 5 rotations on each side.

- Seated Leg Raises: This exercise strengthens the leg muscles without putting stress on the knees. Sit on a sturdy chair with your back straight and feet flat on the floor. Lift one leg straight out in front of you, keeping your knee slightly bent. Hold for a few seconds, then lower your leg back down. Repeat with the other leg. Perform 10 repetitions on each leg.

- Water Aerobics: Exercising in water provides gentle resistance and buoyancy, making it ideal for individuals with arthritis. Consider joining a water aerobics class or performing water exercises in a pool. The water's buoyancy reduces the impact on the joints, allowing for a safe and effective workout.

DIABETES

Diabetes is a condition characterized by high blood sugar levels. Regular exercise can help manage diabetes by improving insulin sensitivity and controlling blood sugar levels. However, it's important to monitor your blood sugar before, during, and after exercise, as it may affect your levels.

Recommended exercises for individuals with diabetes include:

- Brisk Walking: Walking is a low-impact exercise that can be easily incorporated into daily routines. Aim for at least 30 minutes of brisk walking most days of the week. Start with a comfortable pace and gradually increase your speed as you become more fit.

- Yoga: Yoga combines gentle movements, stretching, and deep breathing, making it an excellent choice for individuals with diabetes. It helps improve flexibility, strength, and stress management. Look for beginner-friendly yoga classes or follow along with online videos.

- Resistance Training: Strength training exercises, such as lifting weights or using resistance bands, can help improve insulin sensitivity and build muscle. Start with light weights or resistance and gradually increase as you become stronger.

Remember, it's always important to consult with your healthcare provider before starting any new exercise program, especially if you have a specific health condition. They can provide personalized recommendations and ensure that you exercise safely.

• TRACKING PROGRESS AND MAKING ADJUSTMENTS

In this chapter, we will explore the importance of tracking progress and making adjustments in your balance exercise routine. By monitoring your progress and making necessary adjustments, you can ensure that you are continually challenging yourself and reaping the maximum benefits from your exercises.

WHY TRACKING PROGRESS IS IMPORTANT

Tracking your progress allows you to see how far you've come and provides motivation to keep going. It also helps you identify any areas where you may be struggling or not making as much progress as you'd like. By keeping track of your balance exercises, you can celebrate your achievements and stay committed to your fitness goals.

Tracking your progress also:

- Allows you to identify patterns or trends in your balance improvement
- Helps you set realistic goals and track your progress towards them
- Provides valuable information to share with your healthcare provider or physical therapist
- Allows you to make adjustments to your routine based on your progress

HOW TO TRACK YOUR PROGRESS

There are several ways you can track your progress in your balance exercise routine. Find a method that works best for you and helps you stay motivated.

Here are some options:

- Keep a journal or notebook: Write down the exercises you do each day, along with any notes or observations about your performance. This can help you see improvements over time and identify any areas where you may need to focus more.
- Use a fitness app or wearable device: Many fitness apps and wearable devices allow you to track your exercise routines and monitor your progress. These can provide visual representations of your progress, making it easier to see how far you've come.
- Take photos or videos: If you're comfortable doing so, take photos or videos of yourself performing the exercises. This can be a helpful visual tool to compare your form and balance over time.

MAKING ADJUSTMENTS FOR OPTIMAL RESULTS

As you progress in your balance exercises, it's important to make adjustments to keep challenging yourself. This will help prevent plateaus and ensure that you continue to improve.

Here are some tips for making adjustments:

- Increase the difficulty: Gradually increase the intensity or duration of your exercises as you become more comfortable. For example, you can try holding a balance pose for a few more seconds or adding ankle weights for extra resistance.
- Add variety: Incorporate different exercises or variations of exercises into your routine. This will challenge your balance in new ways and help you continue to improve.
- Seek professional guidance: If you're unsure about how to make adjustments or want personalized advice, consider consulting with a physical therapist or certified fitness professional who specializes in senior fitness.

Remember, it's important to listen to your body and make adjustments that are appropriate for your fitness level and health condition. If you experience any pain or discomfort during exercise, stop and consult with your healthcare provider.

By tracking your progress and making adjustments, you can ensure that you're getting the most out of your balance exercise routine. Stay committed, stay motivated, and enjoy the benefits of improved balance, posture, and confidence!

CHAPTER 12: SUSTAINING YOUR BALANCE JOURNEY

As you continue on your balance journey, it's important to remember that consistency is key. The exercises and routines you've learned in previous chapters are meant to be practiced regularly to yield the best results. In this chapter, we will explore some strategies and tips to help you sustain your commitment to improving your balance, posture, and overall well-being.

SETTING REALISTIC GOALS

When it comes to maintaining an exercise routine, it's crucial to set realistic goals that align with your capabilities and lifestyle. Start by assessing your current fitness level and consider any limitations or health conditions you may have. This will help you establish goals that are both challenging yet attainable.

Important: Remember, it's not about pushing yourself to the limit, but rather making gradual progress over time. By setting achievable goals, you'll be more motivated to continue your balance exercises.

FINDING ACCOUNTABILITY

One of the most effective ways to stay committed to your exercise routine is by finding a source of accountability. This could be a workout buddy, a family member, or even an online community of like-minded individuals. Sharing your progress, challenges, and triumphs with others can provide the support and motivation you need to stay on track.

Important: Having someone to hold you accountable can make all the difference in maintaining your balance journey. Consider finding a partner or joining a group that shares your commitment to improving balance and preventing falls.

ADDING VARIETY

While consistency is important, it's also essential to keep your exercise routine fresh and engaging. Adding variety to your workouts not only prevents boredom but also challenges different muscle groups and improves overall balance.

Important: Try incorporating different exercises from previous chapters into your routine and explore new activities that promote balance, such as yoga or tai chi. This variety will not only keep you motivated but also enhance your progress.

TRACKING YOUR PROGRESS

Tracking your progress is an excellent way to stay motivated and see how far you've come on your balance journey. Consider keeping a journal or using a fitness tracking app to record your workouts, improvements, and any challenges you may encounter.

Important: By documenting your progress, you'll be able to celebrate your achievements and identify areas where you may need additional focus. This self-awareness will help you tailor your exercises to your specific needs and continue making strides in your balance improvement.

STAYING POSITIVE

Maintaining a positive mindset is crucial when it comes to sustaining your balance journey. It's normal to face setbacks or have days when you feel less motivated. However, it's important to remember that every step forward, no matter how small, is progress.

Important: Be kind to yourself and acknowledge the effort you're putting into improving your balance, posture, and overall well-being. Celebrate your achievements, no matter how small, and remember that each day is an opportunity to continue growing stronger.

As you continue on your balance journey, remember that sustaining your commitment is just as important as starting it. Set realistic goals, find accountability, add variety, track your progress, and stay positive. By incorporating these strategies into your daily routine, you'll be well on your way to maintaining your balance, preventing falls, and enjoying an active, independent lifestyle.

• STRATEGIES FOR MAINTAINING BALANCE AND STABILITY OVER TIME

As we age, it becomes increasingly important to prioritize balance and stability in our daily lives. By incorporating simple strategies into our routines, we can improve our overall well-being and reduce the risk of falls. Here are some key strategies to help you maintain balance and stability over time:

1. ENGAGE IN REGULAR PHYSICAL ACTIVITY

Regular physical activity is essential for maintaining balance and stability. Engaging in exercises that focus on strength, flexibility, and coordination can help improve your overall balance. Consider incorporating activities such as walking, swimming, tai chi, or yoga into your routine. These low-impact exercises are gentle on the joints and can help improve muscle strength and flexibility.

2. PRACTICE STANDING ON ONE LEG

Standing on one leg is a simple yet effective exercise for improving balance. Start by standing near a wall or sturdy piece of furniture for support. Lift one leg off the ground and try to balance for 10-15 seconds. Repeat on the other leg. As you become more comfortable, try to increase the duration of the exercise. This exercise helps strengthen the muscles in your legs and improves your ability to maintain balance.

3. INCORPORATE BALANCE EXERCISES INTO YOUR DAILY ROUTINE

Integrating balance exercises into your daily routine is a great way to improve your stability over time. Simple exercises such as heel-to-toe walking, standing on your toes, or marching in place can help strengthen the muscles in your legs and improve your overall balance. Aim to perform these exercises for at least 5 minutes each day.

4. Improve Your Core Strength

A strong core is essential for maintaining balance and stability. Incorporate exercises that target your abdominal muscles, back muscles, and hips into your routine. Planks, bridges, and seated leg lifts are examples of exercises that can help improve your core strength. Consult with a healthcare professional or a certified fitness instructor to ensure you are performing these exercises correctly.

5. Maintain a Healthy Diet

A healthy diet plays a crucial role in maintaining balance and stability. Ensure that you are consuming a well-balanced diet that includes a variety of fruits, vegetables, lean proteins, and whole grains. Adequate intake of vitamins and minerals, particularly calcium and vitamin D, can help support bone health and reduce the risk of osteoporosis.

6. Make Your Home Environment Safe

Creating a safe home environment is essential for preventing falls and maintaining balance. Remove any tripping hazards such as loose rugs or cluttered walkways. Install grab bars in the bathroom and handrails on stairs to provide additional support. Ensure that your home is well-lit, especially in areas prone to falls, such as staircases and hallways.

7. Wear Proper Footwear

The type of footwear you choose can significantly impact your balance and stability. Opt for shoes that provide proper support and have non-slip soles. Avoid wearing high heels or shoes with worn-out soles, as they can increase the risk of falls. Consider consulting with a podiatrist to ensure you are wearing the right footwear for your specific needs.

8. Stay Hydrated

Dehydration can affect your balance and increase the risk of falls. Make sure to drink an adequate amount of water throughout the day to stay hydrated. Aim for at least 8 cups of water per day, or more if you are physically active or live in a hot climate.

By incorporating these strategies into your daily routine, you can improve your balance and stability over time. Remember, consistency is key. Start with small steps and gradually increase the intensity and duration of your exercises. With dedication and perseverance, you can maintain your independence and enjoy an active, confident lifestyle.

• Incorporating Balance Exercises into Daily Lifestyle

As we continue our journey towards better balance and posture, it's important to incorporate balance exercises into our daily lifestyle. By making these exercises a regular part of our routine, we can strengthen our muscles, improve our stability, and reduce the risk of falls. Let's explore some practical ways to integrate balance exercises into our day-to-day activities.

1. Morning Routine

Start your day off on the right foot by incorporating balance exercises into your morning routine. Begin with a simple standing balance exercise:

Stand with your feet hip-width apart, arms relaxed at your sides. Slowly lift one foot off the ground and hold the position for 10 seconds. Repeat with the other foot. Aim for 5 repetitions on each side.

As you get more comfortable with this exercise, challenge yourself by closing your eyes or standing on a pillow for an added balance challenge.

2. Household Chores

Household chores provide an excellent opportunity to work on your balance while completing necessary tasks. Here are a few ideas:

While washing dishes:

- Stand on one leg for 30 seconds, then switch to the other leg.
- Try standing on a cushion or folded towel to create an unstable surface.

While brushing your teeth:

- Stand on your toes for 10 seconds, then lower your heels back down.
- Perform a mini squat by bending your knees slightly and holding the position for 10 seconds.

Remember to always prioritize safety and use support if needed, such as a countertop or chair, to prevent falls while performing these exercises.

3. WALKING BREAKS

During your day, take regular walking breaks to not only improve your cardiovascular health but also enhance your balance. Here's a simple exercise to try:

While walking:

- Take slow, deliberate steps, focusing on lifting your feet off the ground and rolling through each step.
- Try walking on different surfaces, such as grass or gravel, to challenge your balance and engage different muscles.

Remember to wear comfortable shoes with good support and avoid uneven or slippery surfaces to prevent falls.

4. TV TIME

Make the most of your TV-watching sessions by incorporating balance exercises during commercial breaks. Here's a simple exercise to try:

While sitting on the couch:

- Extend one leg out in front of you and hold for 10 seconds, then switch to the other leg.
- Perform ankle circles by rotating your feet clockwise and counterclockwise for 10 seconds each.

These seated exercises help improve ankle strength and flexibility, which are essential for maintaining balance.

By integrating these balance exercises into your daily lifestyle, you'll be taking proactive steps towards improving your balance, posture, and overall well-being. Remember, consistency is key, so aim for at least 5 minutes of balance exercises every day. Stay motivated, stay active, and enjoy the benefits of a stronger, more confident you!

• SEEKING ONGOING SUPPORT AND RESOURCES FOR CONTINUED SUCCESS

Now that you have learned a variety of balance exercises to improve your stability and prevent falls, it is important to seek ongoing support and resources to ensure continued success on your journey towards better balance and posture. By accessing additional tools and guidance, you can enhance your exercise routine and maintain your progress over time.

1. JOIN A SENIOR FITNESS CLASS

One excellent way to receive ongoing support is by joining a senior fitness class. These classes are specifically designed for older adults and often include exercises that target balance and fall prevention. In addition to providing a structured environment for exercise, senior fitness classes offer the opportunity to connect with others who share similar goals and challenges. The camaraderie and support from fellow participants can be incredibly motivating and inspiring.

2. CONSULT WITH A PHYSICAL THERAPIST

If you have specific concerns or medical conditions that affect your balance, it may be beneficial to consult with a physical therapist. A physical therapist can assess your individual needs and create a personalized exercise program tailored to your abilities and goals. They can also provide guidance on proper form and technique to ensure you are performing the exercises correctly and safely.

3. UTILIZE ONLINE RESOURCES

The internet is a vast source of information and resources, and there are many websites and online communities dedicated to senior health and wellness. Explore reputable websites that offer exercise videos, tutorials, and articles specifically targeting balance exercises for seniors. These resources can provide additional guidance and inspiration, allowing you to diversify your exercise routine and keep it fresh and engaging.

4. Engage in Mind-Body Practices

Balance exercises not only benefit your physical well-being but also your mental and emotional well-being. Engaging in mind-body practices such as yoga or tai chi can further enhance your balance, posture, and overall sense of well-being. These practices focus on the connection between the mind and body, incorporating movements, breathing techniques, and mindfulness. Consider attending a local class or using online resources to learn these practices and incorporate them into your routine.

5. Stay Consistent and Motivated

One of the biggest challenges in maintaining an exercise routine is staying consistent and motivated. To overcome this challenge, set realistic goals and create a schedule that works for you. Aim to incorporate balance exercises into your daily routine, even if it's just for a few minutes each day. Celebrate your progress along the way and remind yourself of the benefits you are experiencing, such as improved stability and confidence. Consider finding an accountability partner or joining an online community where you can share your achievements and challenges with others.

Remember, the key to continued success is to stay committed and make balance exercises a regular part of your life. By seeking ongoing support and utilizing available resources, you can maintain your progress and enjoy the long-term benefits of improved balance, posture, and confidence.

Conclusion and Recap of Key Points

As we come to the conclusion of "Balance Exercises for Seniors: 5 minutes a day to improve your balance, posture, and confidence with simple home exercises to fight osteoporosis and prevent falls," it is important to reflect on the key takeaways from this comprehensive guide. Throughout this book, we have explored the importance of maintaining balance and preventing falls as we age, and how simple daily exercises can make a significant impact on our overall well-being.

Recap of Key Points

1. The Impact of Balance: We have learned that balance is not just about physical stability, but also about maintaining our independence and quality of life. By improving our balance, we can enhance our confidence and prevent falls, which are a major concern for seniors.

2. Tailored Exercise Routines: One of the pain points highlighted by many seniors is the lack of exercise resources specifically designed for their needs. This book has provided a solution by offering a tailored exercise regimen that focuses on balance and fall prevention. The exercises are simple, accessible, and can be performed in the comfort of your own home.

3. Empathetic guidance: Throughout this journey I hope I have been your trusted guide, offering empathetic and encouraging advice. I hope with all my heart that my writing style has made you feel as though I have been personally guiding you through each exercise, responding to your concerns, and motivating you to stay committed to your health goals.

4. Safety and Confidence: Fear of injury is a common concern among seniors, especially those with existing health issues like osteoporosis. However, this book has

emphasized safety as a top priority. Detailed step-by-step instructions have been provided for each exercise, ensuring that we can perform them safely and confidently. 5. Commitment and motivation: Committing to an exercise routine can be a challenge, especially if previous attempts have been unsuccessful or if the exercises seem too advanced. I personally have recognized these challenges and provided practical advice on how to stay motivated and incorporate the exercises into our daily routine.

FINAL THOUGHTS

To conclude this book, it is important to remember that improving balance and preventing falls is an ongoing journey. The exercises and guidance provided here are intended to be incorporated into our daily lives, becoming a natural part of our routine. By devoting just five minutes a day to these exercises, we can make a significant difference in our balance, posture and overall well-being. As the professional that I am, I have shared my experience and passion for senior health and wellness in this book, empowering us to take control of our physical health and maintain our independence. With this guide, we can continue to enjoy an active and fulfilling lifestyle without the limitations that imbalances and falls can bring. Remember, the power to improve our balance and quality of life lies within us. Let's make the knowledge and tools provided in this book our own and embark on the journey to better health together.

www.ingramcontent.com/pod-product-compliance
Lightning Source LLC
Chambersburg PA
CBHW081215260726
48653CB00010BA/3658